National Pool and Waterpark Lifeguard/CPR Training

Ellis & Associates, Inc.
Kingwood, Texas

Jeff Ellis
Jill White

JONES AND BARTLETT PUBLISHERS
Sudbury, Massachusetts

Boston   London   Singapore

It is intended that the material contained in this manual will be taught by a licensed National Pool and Waterpark Lifeguard/CPR instructor or by an official instructor in an educational institution. Its use by anyone untrained in NPWLTP teaching methods could result in injury to participants practicing rescue techniques.

Editorial, Sales, and Customer Service Offices
Jones and Bartlett Publishers
40 Tall Pine Drive
Sudbury, MA 01776
(508) 443-5000
(800) 832-0034

Jones and Bartlett Publishers International
Barb House, Barb Mews
London W6 7PA
UK

Library of Congress Cataloging-in-Publication Data

Ellis, Jeffrey L.
    National pool and waterpark lifeguard/CPR training / Jeffrey L.
Ellis, Jill E. White.
        p.   cm.
    Includes index.
    ISBN 0-86720-848-1
    1. Lifeguards—Training of—Handbooks, manuals, etc.   I. White,
Jill E., 1955–   . II. Title.
GV838.72.E45   1994
797.200289—dc20   94-6167
                                                              CIP

Vice President and Publisher: Clayton Jones
Production Editor: Anne Noonan
Manufacturing Buyer: Dana L. Cerrito
Design: Glenna Collett
Editorial Production Service: Progressive Publishing Alternatives
Illustrations: Network Graphics
Typesetting: Omegatype Typography
Cover Design: Marshall Henrichs
Printing and Binding: Banta Company
Cover Printing: John P. Pow Company, Inc.

Printed in the United States of America
98 97 96   10 9 8 7 6 5 4 3

Contents

PART I   LIFEGUARDING SKILLS   1

CHAPTER 1
What Will I Have to Do If I Am Going to See and Recognize an Aquatic Emergency?   3

CHAPTER 2
What Will I Have to Do When I Recognize a Guest in Distress?   21

PART V LIFEGUARD FIRST RESPONDER 119

PART VI PROFESSIONALISM 165

CHAPTER 13
How Will I Be Held Accountable for My Skill Level and Professionalism?   **185**

Do You Meet, Exceed, or Fail Standards?

APPENDICES   **191**

Contributors
Carol L. Fick
Chicago lifeguard course, December 1992
Darby Conover/Wild World Renewal Guards
Denise Fallon
Grant Goold
John Hunsucker, PhD
J. P. Moss/City of Portland
Coy Jones
Bob Logan
Louise Priest
Jack Waterman
Willamalane Park and Recreation District

The following associates of **Ellis & Associates, Inc.** have also contributed greatly to the National Pool and Waterpark Training manuals:

Richard Bleam, Senior Associate
Carol Fick, Vice President
Steve Cable, Senior Associate
Kim Westergaard-Ellis, Secretary/Treasurer
Norm Matzl, Senior Associate
Brenda McVitty, Senior Associate
Joseph Minninger, Senior Associate
Ron Rhinehart, Senior Associate
Chris Stuart, Senior Associate
Terri Adams, Associate
Whitney Matzl, Associate
Mark Oostman, Associate
Vera Solis, Associate
Jill White, Senior Associate

Foreword

Ellis & Associates began development of a lifeguard training program in 1983 to address waterpark safety issues. These efforts led to the development of a state-of-the-art training and risk management program that today includes all types of aquatic facilities and is credited by many national agencies for revolutionizing aquatic safety industry standards in the United States.

The National Pool and Waterpark Lifeguard Training Program has led the industry in:

◆ Developing rescue technology from practitioners of those rescues.

◆ Emphasizing prevention technology by using a national data base to identify high risk populations.

◆ Eliminating body contact rescues and advocating exclusive use of the rescue tube.

◆ Requiring lifeguard accountability by developing operational safety audits and developing the "10/20 Protection Rule" standard of care.

◆ Integrating CPR and lifeguard first responder skills into its lifeguard training curriculum.

◆ Elevating professional lifeguard standards.

◆ Seeking to protect the safety and well-being of professional lifeguards.

◆ Including training in use of bloodborne pathogen devices for aiding guests who are not breathing, bleeding, or in need of CPR.

◆ Bringing pocket mask technology into the water to provide care in the first critical minutes.

Today, because of these innovations, the safety record achieved by our clients continues to remain unmatched by programs of any other national aquatic agency. However, Ellis & Associates believes that lifeguarding is a "dynamic institution" that must remain flexible to address the needs of a rapidly changing profession.

As a result, this textbook reflects the latest and most significant additions to the National Pool and Waterpark Lifeguard Training Program. Our continued commitment to enabling lifeguards to make it work is the basis for our new protocols and instruction format. This process has demanded that we rethink past technology and challenge existing methods to assure that our clients, swimmers, and lifeguards are afforded the highest quality of care available.

The additions to the training program include:

1. A new learner-based, performance-proven instruction format. Skills are taught using methods that integrate many components. This integration results in a teaching sequence that instills confidence and enables effective learning and performance. Decision making, teamwork, communication, and critical thinking skills are core components of this process. Lifeguards will know how to "make it work."

2. New "standard of care" protocols for the protection of National Pool and Waterpark lifeguards who are required to administer rescue breathing and/or CPR. These protocols also enhance the level of care that can be provided to guests.

3. Integration of skills that will prepare lifeguards to manage life-threatening emergency situations they may encounter as a lifeguard first responder.

Additionally, Ellis & Associates is pleased to officially offer this program in the educational market through Jones and Bartlett Publishers, Boston MA. Over the last few years, Ellis & Associates has encountered a growing demand for lifeguarding courses in high schools, vocational/technical schools, colleges and universities. This program allows instructors in the educational market to teach the Ellis & Associates program and makes those students who have been trained by Ellis & Associates approved instructors, eligible for licensure as National Pool and Waterpark lifeguards. Please note that while any instructor may use this text in the classroom, only those instructors who have been previously approved by Ellis & Associates can make their students eligible for licensure as National Pool and Waterpark lifeguards.

In conclusion, Ellis & Associates, Inc. has dedicated itself to improving lifeguard technology and the lifeguard profession. We continue to enjoy a reputation for maintaining the highest standards for service, quality, and accountability available and are proud to release the new National Pool and Waterpark Lifeguard/CPR training course.

Jeff Ellis—Jill White

Acknowledgments

Our firm's service to its clients remains dependent upon the active participation of those who utilize our services and genuinely care to continually improve it. We are convinced that single fact sets us apart from all other national aquatic safety organizations and are proud to enjoy association with such dedicated professionals.

An entire chapter could be devoted to acknowledging the many aquatic safety professionals across this nation who have contributed data, consulted, inspired, and encouraged the development of the material in this textbook. This input from a wide variety of experiences is what continues to make our program a "dynamic institution" that can readily address the needs of a rapidly changing profession. To name everyone would be an impossible task, so we trust that they recognize our sincere appreciation for their assistance by this notation. There are however, several individuals whose contributions need special recognition.

We begin by thanking DoAnn Geiger, Mel and Rosemary Umenhofer, Betty Street, and John Hunsucker whose support enabled my earlier career to grow. Without the confidence and support of Richard Allen, Lamar Parker, Gene Weeks, and Joe Martinez, our group of associates would never have been formed. We also thank Bob, Billie, Gary, Jeff Henry, and Rick and Jana Faber of Schlitterbahn. A special thanks is also expressed to Ron Sutula of Wet N' Wild, Orlando and J. P. Moss of the City of Portland.

We appreciate Gary Maurek, Steve Loose, and Greg Mastriona of the Hyland Hills Park and Recreation District, Tim Demke of the Rockford Park District, Dennis Mattey of the Columbia Association, and Ray Landers of the Deer Park Independent School District for enabling us to diversify our services to the public aquatic community. Further, through the efforts of Steve Cable, Brenda McVitty, Christine Crutcher, and Coy Jones, we were able to begin full program development for the public swimming pool sector.

A special appreciation is also extended to Vera Solis of the College Station Parks and Recreation Department and to Jack and Turk Waterman of Noah's Ark for helping us to understand a staff commitment to excellence.

We appreciate the critical review and support from Tom Werts of Walt Disney World Company as well as a comprehensive review by Dr. Robert D. Clayton and Janis Carley, City of Cape Coral Parks and Recreation, as well as Dean Cerdan, Lee County Parks and Recreation. We also want to thank Walter Johnson and the staff of the National Recreation and Parks Association/Aquatic Section for distributing this textbook and supporting this program. As partners with us, the NRPA and the National Safety Council have chosen to pursue with us the goal of revolutionizing industry standards for aquatic safety in the United States. National Safety Council staff members Donna Siegfried and Neil Boot have been instrumental in the recent changes and growth within our organization.

We are truly indebted to Louise Priest and Grant Goold for their professional expertise and contributions that continue to allow us to reach beyond our present level of knowledge and search for better answers to a wide range of aquatic safety issues.

Most importantly, we thank the thousands of NPWLTP lifeguards who have unselfishly given of their time, expertise, and talent to help make this a practical textbook to benefit their peers. We especially recognize the lifeguards and staff from Dorney Park Wildwater Kingdom for continually providing us a "living laboratory" for research and development of NPWLTP technology.

We give special appreciation to the NPWLTP instructors who have made a commitment to excellence in professional lifeguarding. The continued state-of-the-art training that is being provided by these individuals is what allows the safety record achieved by our clients to remain unmatched by programs of any other national aquatic institution.

Jeff Ellis

Most of the photographs in this textbook were taken during actual facility operation. Many show real rescues and are, therefore, not "technically" perfect. They do, however, accurately illustrate professional lifeguards in the performance of their duties. We thank the client facilities at:

City of Cape Coral	Cape Coral, FL
City of Fife	Fife, WA
City of Raytown	Raytown, MO
Community Recreation Systems	St. Louis, MO
Dorney Park Wildwater Kingdom	Allentown, PA
D.S. Recreational Services	Houston, TX
Enchanted Waves	Federal Way, WA
Fox Valley Park District	Aurora, IL
Naperville Park District	Naperville, IL
Niles Park District	Niles, IL
Noah's Ark	Wisconsin Dells, WI
Oceans of Fun	Kansas City, MO
Raging Waters	San Jose, CA
Rockford Park District	Rockford, IL
Splashtown USA	Spring, TX
Splish Splash	Riverhead, NY
Wet N' Wild	Arlington, TX

Introduction

Course Overview

Professional lifeguards prevent drownings. If lifeguards don't perform, someone will die.

Last year alone, National Pool and Waterpark lifeguards made over 19,000 documented rescues. In each instance, if the lifeguard had not intervened, the situation would have resulted in a drowning.

The National Pool and Waterpark Lifeguard Training Program (NPWLTP) provides professional lifeguard training as one of the core components of a comprehensive aquatic safety system. This program and system, developed and managed by Ellis & Associates, Inc. (E & A), protects swimmers and lifeguards from catastrophic injury and drowning.

This course is designed for a highly skilled and responsible individual and will help prepare you for one of the most challenging jobs you will ever have. Few other positions carry the responsibility to **guard, protect,** and **save human lives.**

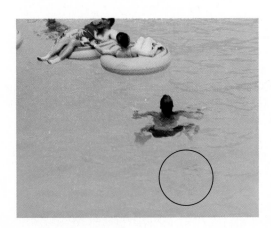

The lifeguard has the responsibility to guard, protect, and save human life. Few other positions carry this level of responsibility.

The purpose of the course is to equip you with the skills and technical knowledge to become an effective member of your aquatic facility team. Licensure as an NPWL trained lifeguard shows that you and other lifeguards employed by your facility have participated in levels of training extending beyond the reasonable standard.

For personnel at waterparks, this training is of particular value because it includes rescue techniques specifically designed for use in waves and currents.

It is intended that the material contained in this manual will be taught by an approved National Pool and Waterpark lifeguard instructor or by an official instructor in an educational institution. Its use by anyone untrained in NPWL teaching methods could result in injury to participants practicing rescue techniques.

The National Pool and Waterpark Lifeguard Training Program is divided into the following training courses:

- Shallow water lifeguard training.

- Pool lifeguard training.

- Special facilities lifeguard training.

Your training course will be unlike any lifeguard training you may have had before. Some of the skills in the course include:

- How to anticipate how incidents will occur.

- How to recognize incidents.

- How to manage an incident with skills that work.

- How to think critically about complications that real situations might present.

- How to be professional.

- How to protect your safety and well-being.

You must be able to react and make a rescue work without having to think about how to perform the various parts. This course will give you that confidence. In class, you will learn how to manage situations by simulating the "real deal" as closely as possible. You will learn skills that work, are safe, and are practical.

As a professional lifeguard, you will have two primary responsibilities:

- Prevent drowning/accidents.

- Provide rescue and emergency care.

At this point you may want to examine what you really think about lifeguarding, and how you view the job as a lifeguard. Is it "fun in the sun" all day?

If you believe lifeguarding is a fun job that offers time to "take it easy" and "get that beautiful tan," you might want to select another job. Let's face it, most lifeguards are athletic, physically attractive, active young people. It is fair to say that the public has this image of today's lifeguard.

Having a job with such "status" among peers could tempt you to concentrate on the wrong people and places when lifeguarding. If you think this job will give you the opportunity to watch many good looking people, you are right. However, if you let yourself become dominated by such interests while you are supposed to be protecting swimmers, it could be the most tragic mistake you ever make. It is common for the glamour associated with lifeguarding to wear off within 2 or 3 days after you begin working and you discover what lifeguarding is truly about.

If you decide to proceed, and if you do successfully complete the training and are employed as a lifeguard, it will undoubtedly become one of the most challenging, yet rewarding, jobs you will ever experience.

Course Information

The following chart outlines the various National Pool and Waterpark Lifeguard course requirements.

- Facility where license is valid:

   Shallow water lifeguard: Any client facility where water is 4 feet deep or less.

   Pool lifeguard: Any client pool of any depth that has not been classified as a special facility by Ellis & Associates.

   Special facilities lifeguard: Any client facility that has been classified as a "special facility" by Ellis & Associates.

- Minimum age to obtain license/number of years valid:

   Shallow water lifeguard: 15/1 year

   Pool lifeguard: 15/1 year

   Special facilities lifeguard: 16/1 year

- Prerequisite skills, swim distance using crawl or breaststroke without resting:

   Shallow water lifeguard: 50 yds

   Pool lifeguard: 100 yds

   Special facilities lifeguard: 200 yds

- Prerequisite skills, surface dive, and bring up a 10-pound brick and bring it to the wall from a depth of:

   Shallow water lifeguard: 4 ft (must also swim a distance of 10 ft underwater)

   Pool lifeguard: 8 ft

   Special facilities lifeguard: 8 ft

- Prerequisite skills, treading water without using hands for:

   Shallow water lifeguard: None

   Pool lifeguard: 1 minute

   Special facilities lifeguard: 2 minutes

◆ **Qualifications for license renewal:**

All courses: Meet all prerequisites for the regular course.

Attend review/update class.

Pass written and water practical examination.

◆ **Course rules:**

All courses: Enter the water feet first at **all** times.

When using a rescue tube, keep it between yourself and the victim.

Wear hat, sunscreen, and sunglasses if outdoors.

◆ **General course information:**

1. All courses include National Safety Council CPR (*Journal of the American Medical Association*/American Heart Association standards) Certification for Adult, Child and Infant, and include Lifeguard First Responder first aid skills.

2. If you do not pass all of the requirements for the course you are taking, you must take the **entire course** again to be considered for licensure. (If you do not pass the requirements in a review course, you must enroll in the full course to be considered for licensure.)

◆ **General information about the NPWLTP license:**

1. Any license becomes valid only when you:

Meet prerequisites.

Pass all practical (water and CPR) tests.

Pass all written tests with an 80% score.

Demonstrate proper attitude, maturity, and judgment.

Complete site-specific training at your facility.

Your license is subject to revocation at any time. Read the license agreement carefully before you sign it to be sure you understand your responsibilities.

2. Educational Market:

Students successfully completing a training course taught by an Ellis & Associates approved instructor in an educational institution, (high school, vocational/technical, colleges and universities) are eligible to receive licensure as National Pool and Waterpark Lifeguards. Students can obtain a license request form from their instructor. This form needs to be completed by the student and also verified by the instructor. The completed form should be submitted along with the appropriate registration fee to the following address for processing:

License Request Department
Ellis & Associates
3506 Spruce Park Circle
Kingwood, TX 77345

Please allow three to four weeks for processing.

Lifeguarding Skills

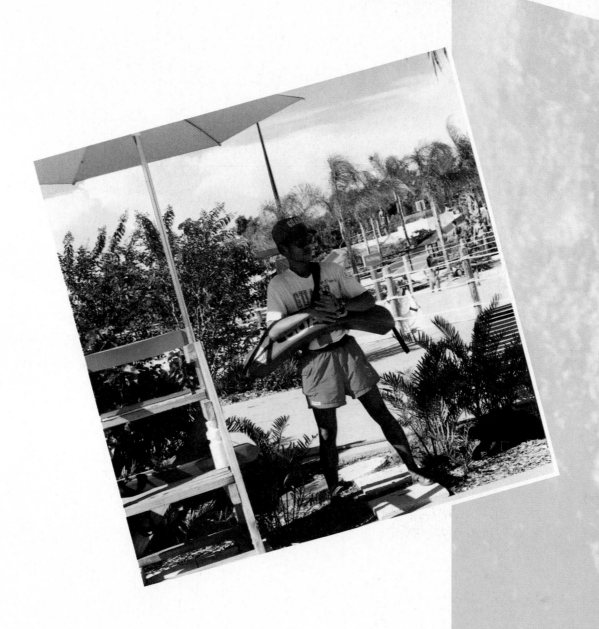

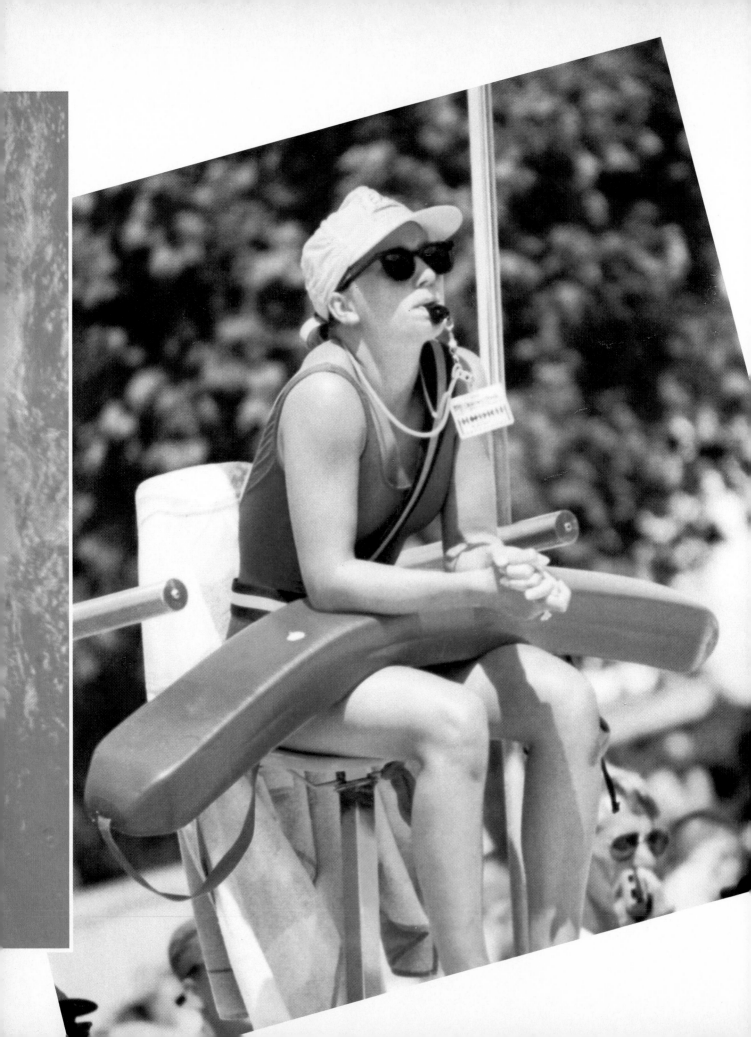

What Will I Have to Do If I Am Going to See and Recognize an Aquatic Emergency?

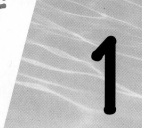

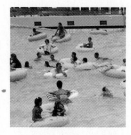

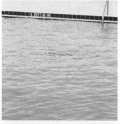

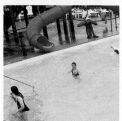

CHAPTER OBJECTIVES

After completing the chapter and related water work, the lifeguard candidate should be able to:

1. Understand and implement the 10/20 Protection Rule.
2. Demonstrate the four scanning patterns and understand the importance of diligence.
3. Describe the two types of drowning and characteristics of each.
4. Identify high risk groups, locations, and times.
5. Rotate without loss of eye contact to the zone.

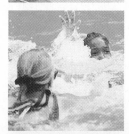

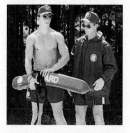

Consider how you will actually spend your time as a lifeguard. Almost ALL your time will be spent **lifeguarding,** not rescuing. And there is more to lifeguarding than just sitting in the chair.

You need to know what to do with your time to be a professional lifeguard. You need to know how to watch, where to watch, what to look for, and how to stay alert every second. This chapter will describe the techniques that are the most critical for you to master in your training as a professional lifeguard.

THE 10/20 PROTECTION RULE

The National Pool and Waterpark Lifeguard Training Program is based on the 10/20 Protection Rule. It has been proven that if an aquatic incident involving a guest in distress can be managed within the first 30 seconds, it can be prevented from becoming a catastrophic event that might possibly result in a drowning. The 10/20 Protection Rule means that you must be able to detect distress within the first 10 seconds, and then you have 20 seconds to reach the guest and render aid.

Any decision about staffing, guard locations, or safety concerns should always be made by asking, "Can the 10/20 Protection Rule be followed in this situation?" The only facilities not required to use the 10/20 Protection Rule at all times are protected lakefront, open water, or other special areas, which are subject to the 3-minute rule. In addition to scanning the zone every 10 seconds, the entire lakefront area must be able to be searched within 3 minutes. This rule is described in more detail in Chapter 12.

ZONES

When lifeguarding, you will have a specific area assigned to you that is your "**zone.**" This will be your area of responsibility, and it will be different for each guard station at your facility.

In order to maintain the 10/20 Protection Rule, you **must** be able to look at every position of your zone every 10 seconds. For you to physically do this:

1. You must be able to scan the area every 10 seconds. The zone cannot be so large that it takes you longer than 10 seconds to see everything.
2. You cannot be distracted for even a second, or some part of your zone will not be scanned.
3. You must be able to swim to the furthest area of your zone within 20 seconds.

DILIGENCE

You must constantly avoid distractions while lifeguarding. Lifeguarding can be routine and boring—staring at water is not particularly exciting. For example, try filling your bathtub with water, pulling up a chair, and watching the water for 1/2 hour. It seems almost impossible to sit and stare at it for 30 minutes. Staring at water in a pool, even an empty pool, can be as bad. Pretend you have no guests in your pool, only flat, calm water, yet you must look at it, scan it, constantly.

Keep your eyes on the water!

Now let's put a roller coaster on the other side of the pool.

Keep your eyes on the water!

Between the pool and the roller coaster add two very attractive young men and young women lying on the grass in very brief bathing suits.

Keep your eyes on the water!

Add crowd noise and a loud source of music; you can barely hear yourself talk.

Keep your eyes on the water!

A mother walks up to you and begins complaining because her child cannot hang onto the wall while the waves are on.

Keep your eyes on the water!

Add a blazing hot summer sun, a dry throat, and an uneasy stomach. You cannot become distracted even for a few seconds. The job is tough and demanding, and there can be no compromise.

Not compromising, no matter what the circumstances, is known as diligence. It is one of the most important characteristics you can develop as a professional lifeguard.

SCANNING

As you diligently watch your zone, your eyes need to move in regular patterns to be sure you look at each area. This eye movement is known as scanning.

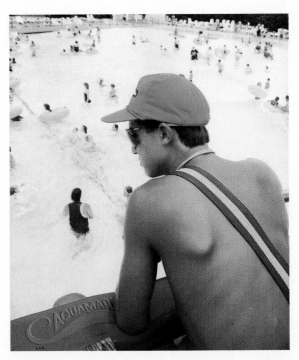

Remember the 10/20 Protection Rule at all times.

You will develop your own techniques for scanning that work best for you. Here are some suggestions from experienced lifeguards:

1. Know the exact geographical area to be scanned and develop a pattern for scanning it.

2. Know where your area overlaps with another lifeguard's area. Know this for each guard position at your facility.

3. Time your scanning so that every area is checked every 10 seconds—this means your whole area, not just where the "action" is.

4. Know which parts of your zone are high risk or blind spots and allow more time for scanning these areas.

5. Ask the lifeguard you are replacing if there are any special circumstances you should know about.

6. Be able to interrupt the scan to check high risk areas such as slide entrances or diving boards to make sure anyone entering the water is able to make it safely to the side or shallow water.

7. Do not forget that the pool is three-dimensional—scan from the bottom up, then across the surface.

Each facility should have a basic chart describing the scanning areas for each guarding position. However, most facilities adjust the scanning area based on the number of swimmers in the pool. You should know the scanning area for each guarding position. For example, if there are eight guarding positions, you should know the adjustments for each area.

If the facility adjusts the normal guarding zone areas when the pool is very crowded, then you are required to know the eight areas for crowded conditions in addition to the eight normal scanning areas. If the facility also eliminates some guarding positions when the pool is less crowded, you must also know that coverage. This could mean that you could be responsible for knowing 24 guard zones, depending on where you are guarding, the condition of the pool, and the number of swimmers.

The top figure on page 7 shows a standard wave pool that uses two chairs on each side, has two standing lifeguards where the waves break, has one lifeguard in the shallow water, and has one lifeguard on the bulkhead. Each lifeguard's area is designated by an arc. Assume that this diagram is for a normal swimmer load at this particular wave pool. Notice that almost every area of the pool is scanned by two lifeguards. In some cases three lifeguards overlap the same area. The area where the waves break and the deep end of the pool both have double coverage.

The next diagram highlights the scanning areas for lifeguards 5 and 8. On a slow day the pool may choose not to have lifeguard position 1 filled. Look at how this could affect the coverage of the pool unless the scanning zones are changed.

The shaded area in the next diagram now has single lifeguard coverage, and it is the deep end, where we know statistically that a high number of rescues occur. Suppose lifeguard 2 or 8 must make a swimming rescue. Who should cover this area? Also, notice that if either lifeguard 3 or 7 must make a rescue, the backup by other lifeguards

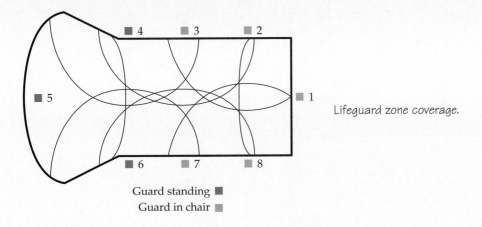

Lifeguard zone coverage.

Guard standing ■
Guard in chair ■

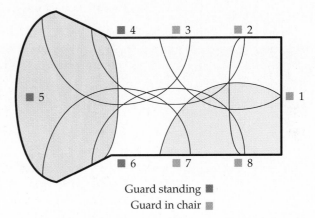

Lifeguard zone coverage, lifeguards 5 and 8.

Guard standing ■
Guard in chair ■

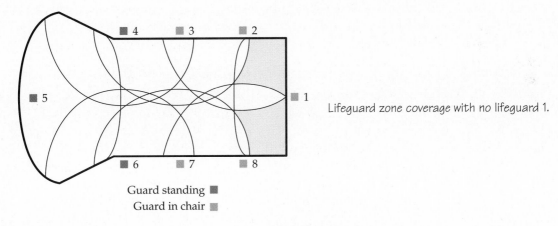

Lifeguard zone coverage with no lifeguard 1.

Guard standing ■
Guard in chair ■

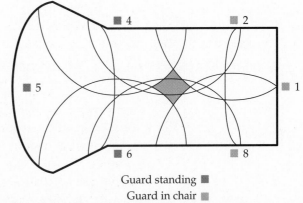

Lifeguard zone coverage, no lifeguards 3 or 7.

Guard standing ■
Guard in chair ■

appears to be adequate. However, look at what happens if you remove both of these lifeguards.

The shaded area is not covered if both lifeguards 3 and 7 are involved in a rescue. Obviously, other lifeguards can easily adjust their scanning areas to cover for the lifeguards who are missing. As the situation changes in your facility, so must your scanning.

It does not matter if you identify your scanning zone as a rectangle or as a semicircle. If your pool better lends itself to setting up a rectangular pattern, that's fine. The important point is to overlap areas, not miss any portion of the pool, and develop a scanning technique that works for you. The next figures show some suggested scanning patterns you could try that will allow you to cover a zone like the one pictured every 10 seconds. Let your eyes follow the direction of the arrows. Remember to choose a scanning technique that you feel comfortable with.

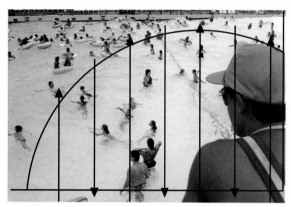
Scanning pattern: up and down.

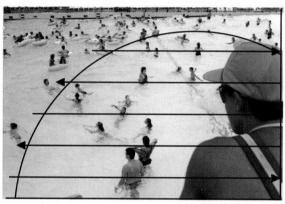
Scanning pattern: side to side.

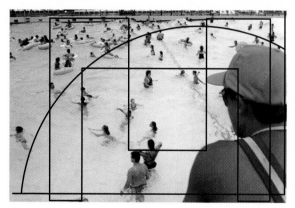
Scanning pattern: geometric.

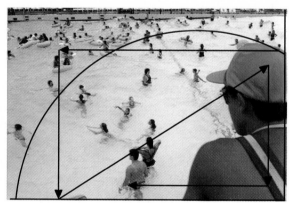
Scanning pattern: double triangle.

You can also change your scanning pattern at any time. Changing your pattern occasionally is one method of maintaining your diligence and attention every second you are on duty as a lifeguard.

Another addition to your scanning pattern that is particularly helpful if the water is cloudy, there is surface glare, or you find your concentration hard to maintain is to count the guests in your zone as you scan.

Obviously, this technique would not be appropriate if your zone was filled with a large number of guests, but it is effective with smaller numbers of guests.

What Are You Looking for When You Scan?

A person in distress will fall into one of three categories, each with its own characteristics, based on location in the pool. Persons in distress will be:

1. On the surface, either conscious or unconscious.
2. Just below the surface (within arms' reach) either conscious or unconscious.
3. Below the surface (beyond arms' reach) either conscious or unconscious.

When you scan, you are looking for:

◆ **Location:** Is the distressed guest on the surface, within arms' reach or below arms' reach?

◆ **Condition:** Is the distressed guest conscious or unconscious?

Victims in each category will show behavior that will alert you to the fact that they are in distress in the water. People in trouble in the water look different from those around them:

1. Their **eyes** may be opened **wide** or tightly shut.
2. Their **bodies** may be stiff and **tense.**

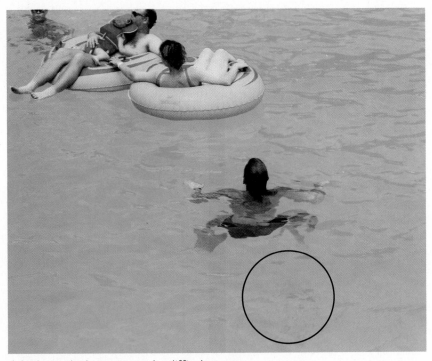

A body on the bottom may be difficult to see.

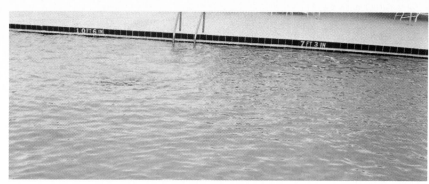

A body on the bottom may be difficult to see.

3. Conscious victims are usually in a **diagonal** or **vertical** position in the water.

4. Their **arms** may **flail** up and down or reach and grab.

5. Their **heads** are generally **back,** with their mouths gasping for air.

6. They usually show **no leg movement.**

7. They are usually **disoriented.**

8. They may be unconscious (**limp** or **rigid**).

9. There may be **no body movement.**

10. They may be trying to grab an object to get support (lane line, inner tube, or another guest).

A guest in distress on top of the water will be noticed easier than a guest in distress under the water. This is one reason you need to get into the habit of scanning from the bottom to the surface.

What will a body under the water, or on the bottom, look like? The general perception is that in a clear pool a body on the bottom will show up clearly, and you will be able to see it immediately. However, studies show that a body on the bottom is not easily visible and depending on the number of guests in the water, the disturbance of the water, glare, and reflection, a body may be almost impossible to see. This is why it is so important to include the bottom in your scan. Pay particular attention to dark, tiled, or painted areas.

When water clarity and crowd conditions allow—guard from the bottom up. A body on the bottom may look only like a blurred spot. If you notice any change in the bottom of the pool and cannot immediately determine what it is, **find out. If you don't know . . . go!**

Any movement, **or lack of movement,** that is out of the ordinary will also demand your immediate attention, quick evaluation, and appropriate response. The faster you can recognize that a guest is in distress, the more effective your management of the incident will be.

Be prepared for any type of situation. Something as simple as a guest trying to stand up from a face-down floating position could turn into a drowning. Inexperienced swimmers have a very difficult time with this skill and could literally drown because they could not stand or lost their balance while trying to stand. Your diligence and attention to detail and movement patterns will prevent drownings.

DROWNING AND IMMERSION

An understanding of the factors involved in the drowning process will also help you recognize when an individual is in distress and is quickly becoming a drowning victim. There are two types of drowning: wet and dry.

Wet Drowning

Wet drowning is death caused by a fluid in the lungs. Drowning victims usually follow a pattern of reactions or five stages of the drowning process. Be aware, however, that there is always the possibility that your distressed guest will have conditions or a situation that will not follow the stage pattern. For example, a distressed guest who suffers a heart attack and quickly slips under the water will not ever exhibit symptoms of the first two stages. Drownings in the water include the following stages:

1. Surprise (10–20 seconds). Distressed guests recognize the danger and are afraid, are usually in a diagonal or vertical position, will probably not be kicking or using their legs, will be moving their arms at or near the surface in random "grasping" or "flapping" motions, will have the head tilted back, face upwards, and may, **or may not,** be making any sounds. Usually, people who are drowning are too busy trying to get air to call for help.

2. Involuntary breath holding. In this second stage, victims may continue to struggle, usually make no sound, are not breathing, because the muscles have taken over the breathing process and are not under conscious control, and will become unconscious in about 90 seconds.

3. Unconscious (60 seconds). In this stage, the victims will not move their arms or legs, will sink to the bottom, either slowly or rapidly, depending on factors such as the amount of air left in their lungs, body weight, and density, etc., and will remain unconscious (and die) unless breathing and circulation are reestablished by rescue breathing and/or CPR.

4. Hypoxic convulsions. In this fourth stage, victims may look like they are having a convulsion, due to lack of oxygen in the brain, may appear rigid or stiff, may jerk violently and/or froth at the mouth, and will remain unconscious (and die) unless breathing and circulation are restored after the convulsions subside by rescue breathing and/or CPR.

5. Clinical death. Clinical death usually follows if breathing and circulation are not reestablished within the first 3 minutes after immersion. Even if CPR efforts are successful at the scene, many drowning victims die as a result of secondary complications. This is another reason why it is so important to activate the Emergency Medical Services system and get advanced life support to a drowning victim as quickly as possible.

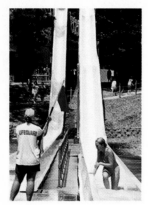

High velocity activities have a potential for dry drowning.

Children seem to move much more quickly through the stages of drowning and often never clearly exhibit the symptoms of the first stages of drowning. Their pattern of distress is usually one of a slight struggle while they are completely submerged, followed immediately by unconsciousness. The child may appear to be "bobbing" underwater in an attempt to get to the surface.

Dry Drowning

Dry drowning victims asphyxiate (suffocate) as a result of a laryngospasm. There is no water in the lungs of the victim. Asphyxiation is caused when droplets of water irritate the epiglottis, which then closes over the glottis, preventing air from entering the air passage.

The following definitions may help your understanding of dry drowning:

- The **larynx** is the upper part of the trachea where the vocal cords are located.

- A **spasm** is an involuntary and abnormal muscular contraction.

- The **epiglottis** is cartilage, behind the tongue and in front of the glottis, which works somewhat like a valve, normally up (open) when a person is breathing, but down (closed over the glottis) when swallowing or in a spasm.

- The **glottis** is the opening and/or elongated space between vocal folds.

Dry drowning generally occurs with activities in which water has the opportunity to enter the mouth at a high velocity, such as speed slides, dives off a diving board, or slides that end in a free fall from a height. In a dry drowning, the victim:

1. May at first have a choking or gagging reaction.

2. May show violent choking and/or gagging.

3. May go into a laryngospasm as long as 10 minutes after the initial reaction.

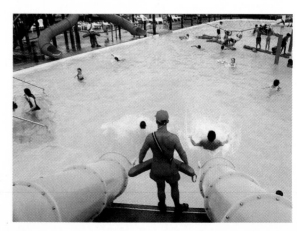

High velocity activities have a potential for dry drowning.

DROWNING COMPARISON

Wet Drowning	Dry Drowning
◆ Accounts for approximately 80% of drownings.	Accounts for approximately 20% of drownings.
◆ Occurs because the victim aspirates (draws by suction) water into the lungs.	Occurs because the victim asphyxiates (suffocates) due to laryngospasm.
◆ Usually causes death in 3–6 minutes from immersion.	Onset usually occurs in 6–10 minutes after the water droplet irritation.
◆ Victims are in the water.	Victims may or may not be in the water.
◆ Rescue procedures range from in-water rescue to full CPR.	Procedure is to rescue (if in water) and/or assess airway, breathing and circulation as taught in CPR. (Chapter 5)

Now that you know what to look for so that you can tell that a guest is in distress, you also need to be aware of high risk situations that will allow you to anticipate potential incidents before they occur.

HIGH RISK CONCERNS

There are three high risk concerns:

1. High risk guests: guests who are at high risk of becoming distressed.
2. High risk locations: places where guests are more likely to become distressed.
3. High risk times: times of the day that have statistically had the highest rescue rates.

All of the high risk categories have been determined by actual **rescue statistics** involving more than 90 million guests, and 55,000 documented rescues compiled by Ellis & Associates.

High Risk Guests: Who Are They?

High risk guests include the following groups:

1. **Children between the ages of 7 and 12** because they are smaller, not very strong, have less skill in the water, and are less aware of danger.
2. **Non swimmers or poor swimmers** because they may have had less opportunity to gain aquatic experience.

3. **Parents with small children** because they may not have enough swimming skill to support both themselves and their child/children.

4. **Intoxicated guests** because even one drink slows down reactions and the ability to control movement, balance, and judgment.

5. **People with unusual or extreme body proportions** because their bodies will react differently in the water than other guests.

6. **Guests wearing lifejackets** because the lifejacket may not fit properly or may not hold the guest up, or the guest may not be used to the feeling of wearing the lifejacket and may panic.

7. **The elderly** because they may tire easily or have medical conditions that prevent them from having the strength or mobility of their younger years.

8. **Disabled guests** because they may be unfamiliar with how your facility will affect their abilities to move.

9. **Guests wearing clothes** because the clothes absorb water, become heavy, and make movement more difficult. Also, if a guest does not have a bathing suit, it may indicate a low experience level.

10. **Every guest** because an unexpected aquatic incident can happen to **anyone,** regardless of swimming ability or experience.

High Risk Locations

Most guests get into trouble:

1. In deep water.
2. In wave pools, especially at the swell/break depth of about 5 feet.
3. In activity pools, especially exiting from slides.
4. In slide catch pools, where water is 4 feet or less.
5. In hydraulic currents of whitewater inner tube rides.
6. In return currents along sides of wave pools.
7. In diving tanks or other deep water pools.
8. In pools where there is a stair, a drop off, a ladder, or a slide.
9. In a lake beyond the life lines, around or between piers and docks.

High Risk Times

Times when most guests get into distress in the water are:

1. Midday, between 12 and 4 p.m.
2. Anytime during crowded conditions.

As a professional lifeguard, you now know where to look, what to look for, and how to look. While you are on duty, you know the importance of **diligence** and will maintain the 10/20 Protection Rule at all times.

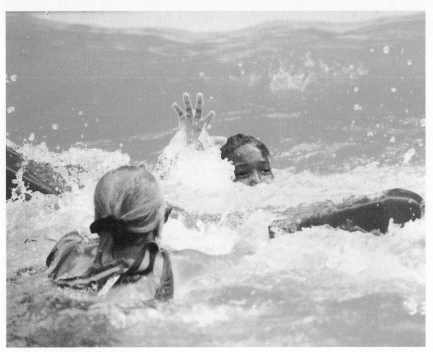

Rescuing a high risk guest.

LIFEGUARD ROTATIONS

What happens when it is time to leave your post and be relieved by another lifeguard? Your system of **rotation** is very important to be sure that the 10/20 Protection Rule is maintained at a time when it is very easy to become distracted.

For maximum zone protection and professionalism, conduct your rotation in the following manner:

1. Incoming lifeguard reports to station.

2. Equipment is transferred.

3. Incoming lifeguard watches zone.

4. Equipment is transferred.

5. Outgoing lifeguard watches zone.

6. Equipment is transferred.

7. Rotation is complete as outgoing lifeguard leaves.

As you rotate:

- Always walk to the lifeguard station.

- Be timely.

- Limit the conversation to facts about the swimmers in the zone.

- Remember guests are aware of your movements and how you conduct yourself.

- Be sure the incoming guard is ready and has assumed responsibility before you leave.

Rotate professionally with no loss of eye contact to the zone.

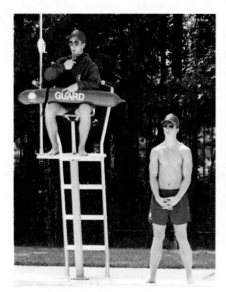

Incoming guard reports.

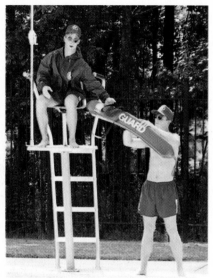

Transfer equipment and responsibility for zone.

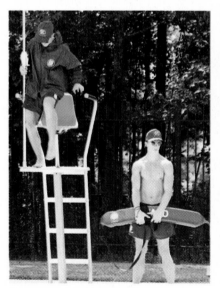

Outgoing guard leaves chair.

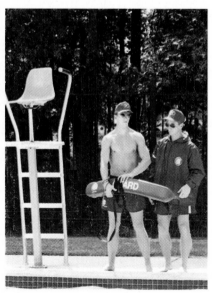

Transfer equipment and responsibility for zone back to outgoing guard.

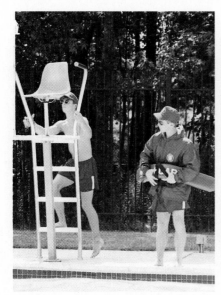

Incoming guard enters chair; outgoing guard scans zone.

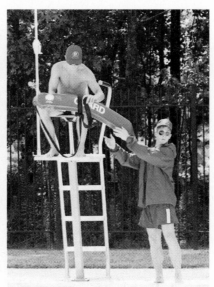

Transfer equipment.

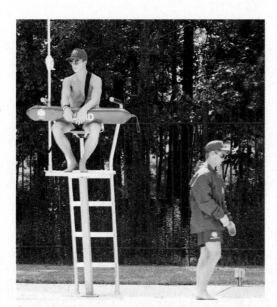

Outgoing lifeguard leaves only after incoming guard is ready and has assumed zone responsibility.

REVIEW QUESTIONS

1. What water depth differentiates a shallow water facility from a deep water facility? _____ feet.

2. The NPWLTP license is good for _____ year(s).

3. List three important areas that the NPWLTP course emphasizes.

   a.

   b.

   c.

4. T   F   Dry drowning occurs more frequently than wet drowning.

5. T   F   To "aspirate" means to "suffocate."

6. T   F   The rescue procedure for someone experiencing a laryngospasm would include assessing the ABC's as taught in CPR.

7. T   F   Guests experiencing dry drowning may or may not be in the water.

8. T   F   Children may experience the stages of wet drowning much more quickly than adults.

9. Name three guests who would be considered high risk.

   a.

   b.

   c.

10. What is the leading cause of injury at a facility? _____

11. Most rescues occur at what time of day? _____

12. T   F   All swimmers are at risk at your facility.

13. T   F   A guest on the bottom will be easy to see.

14. T   F   Guests can be conscious on the bottom and still need rescuing.

15. T   F   Scanning patterns for a zone should never be changed.

16. T   F   When rotating it is important to look professional and maintain the 10/20 Protection Rule.

17. The 10/20 Protection Rule allows you _____ seconds to see and recognize an aquatic emergency, and _____ seconds to perform a rescue and begin management of the situation.

18. T   F   You should focus on and scan the location of the guests in your facility.

SKILL SHEET 1

Scanning and Rotation

1

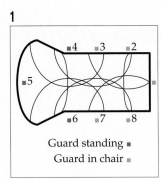

Know your zone.

2

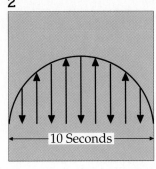

Scan zone every 10 seconds.

3

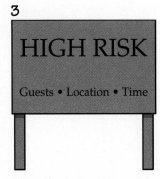

Watch for high risk groups, locations, time.

4

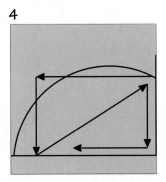

Have a scanning pattern.

5

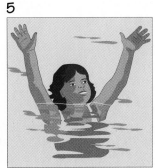

Know distress symptoms.

6

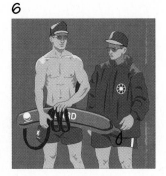

Rotate professionally.

KEY POINTS:

- ◆ Never compromise diligence.
- ◆ Complete rotations while maintaining the 10/20 Protection Rule.
- ◆ Change scanning patterns occasionally.

CRITICAL THINKING:

1. What do you do if the guard on your right blows one long whistle blast and is going to make a rescue?

2. What are some situations that would change your scanning?

3. How does the 10/20 Protection Rule affect what you do?

4. What circumstances might make it more difficult for you to remain diligent? How can you control them?

5. What can you do to keep your attention level up no matter what the circumstances?

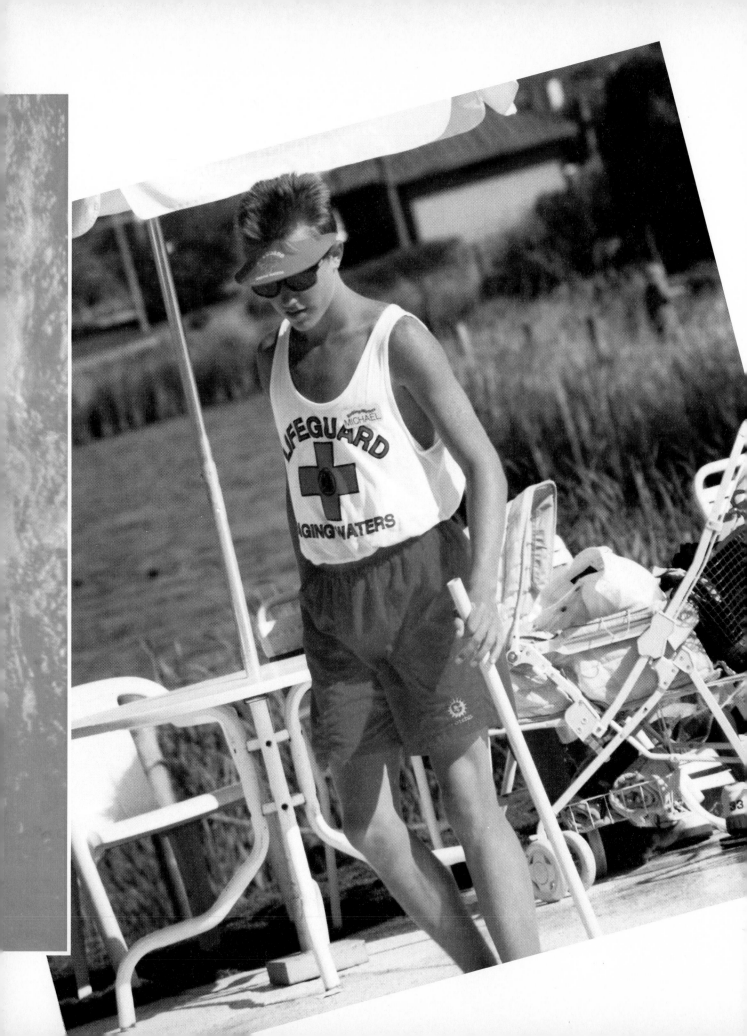

What Will I Have to Do When I Recognize a Guest in Distress?

CHAPTER

2

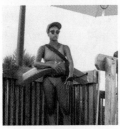

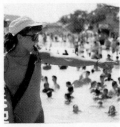

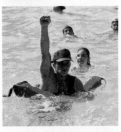

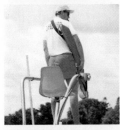

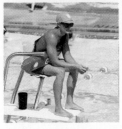

CHAPTER OBJECTIVES

After completing the chapter and related water work, the lifeguard candidate should be able to:

1. Activate the Emergency Action System.
2. Demonstrate seven lifeguard communication skills.
3. Understand the concept of team lifeguarding.
4. Identify the differences between an assist and a rescue.
5. Recognize the importance of non-body-contact rescues and the use of the rescue tube.

When you recognize an aquatic emergency, you will respond in a way that will begin a chain of events that will help you and your fellow lifeguards handle the situation in the best manner possible. This chain of events is called the Emergency Action System (EAS), and it is a plan designed specifically for your facility.

Your aquatic facility will have this plan in writing, and it explains the role of each member of the aquatic team in an emergency. You need to read, discuss, and **practice** the plan. The EAS covers all kinds of emergencies.

The EAS should always be activated by the lifeguard who recognizes the emergency, and it is done by blowing your whistle in one long blast. The activation of the EAS means that more than one lifeguard's attention is required for assistance, rescue, and/or emergency care. Even if you do not need help with the actual rescue, you need to let other lifeguards know you are making a rescue so they can watch your zone and be ready to assist.

BASIC PRINCIPLES OF THE EMERGENCY ACTION SYSTEM

Lifeguard on Rescuer's Left Covers Both Zones

The lifeguard to the immediate left of the whistling guard always covers the rescuer's area and serves as the backup lifeguard. If the rescuing lifeguard needs help the left lifeguard will be the one to assist.

This also means that **you** are the backup for any lifeguards stationed to your right. You need to be prepared at all times to cover their zone if they go in for a rescue and to assist if the lifeguard signals for help.

If Two or More Lifeguards Are Rescuing, Close the Activity

Other staff members will begin to clear the facility of remaining swimmers. When two or more lifeguards are required for a rescue, the activity must be closed until the emergency has passed and the lifeguards have returned to their stations.

COMMUNICATION

Crowd noise, weather, acoustics, and distance can all make communication difficult at an aquatic facility. You must be able to communicate with guests to enforce rules, and you must also be able to communicate with fellow lifeguards and supervisors to get assistance and keep your operation running smoothly.

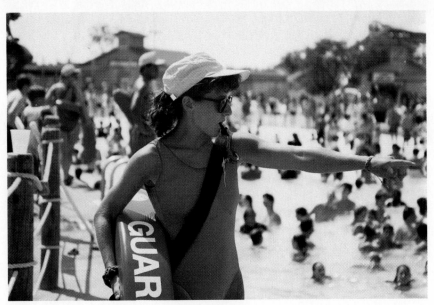

Good communication skills are essential for the professional lifeguard.

Whistle and hand signals are good ways to communicate. Many fa-cilities also use telephones, walkie-talkies, megaphones, or other com-munication devices.

Whistles

Your whistle will be your most frequently used piece of communication equipment. It is required that you have a whistle with you at all times while on duty.

Use a whistle in good working order with a shrill tone that cuts through crowd noise. Whistles are to be blown **loudly** and **firmly.** The following whistle signals will allow you to control your area and com-municate several different types of situations to your fellow lifeguards or supervisors. In addition to, or in place of these standard signals, your facility may choose to develop its own communication system. For ex-ample, verbal and numerical codes are used frequently in indoor facili-ties where whistles are too loud for anything other than activating the Emergency Action System.

You need to know, **and practice,** the communication signals used in your facility.

One Short Blast.   Use one short whistle blast to gain a guest's atten-tion. After you get the guest's attention, it is best if you use hand signals and speak clearly if you need to give him further instructions. If practi-cal, take off your sunglasses when speaking directly to a guest.

Two Short Blasts.   Use two short whistle blasts to gain another life-guard's attention. As you blow two short blasts, raise your hand or tap the top of your head. This way, your fellow lifeguards or the supervisor can quickly know which lifeguard has whistled.

One Long Blast.   Use one long whistle blast to activate the Emergency Action System. This indicates that you are going to do a rescue. Usually this means that you are entering the water, and that other members of your lifeguard team must become involved.

If you are working at a wave pool, you should also hit the emergency stop button (E-stop) before entering the water. The lifeguard to your left covers your zone (in addition to her own). In a wave pool or slide, this lifeguard is also responsible for making sure the waves or dispatch has been stopped. A head lifeguard or supervisor should respond to all water rescues whenever possible or practical, as a rescue report must be completed after all water rescues.

Two Long Blasts.   Use two long whistle blasts to indicate a major emergency. This communicates the need for two or more lifeguards, and the aquatic activity must be immediately closed and cleared of swimmers. The lifeguards not involved in rescue attempts are responsible for securing the pool before providing additional support to the rescuing lifeguards.

Hand Signals

Hand signals are primarily used with whistles to help communicate. Hold hand signals for 5 seconds when possible, to make sure they are noticed.

Pointing.   Pointing is used to give direction. It can be used along with one short whistle blast to indicate to guests what you would like them to do. You can point, along with two short whistle blasts, to communicate with another lifeguard or your supervisor. This is especially helpful when you would like to point out a high risk guest.

Raised Clenched Fist.   A raised clenched fist means you need help. It might be accompanied by two short whistle blasts if you were at the side of the pool, on deck, or in your chair. It would not be accompanied by a whistle if you were in the water. (Remember, the lifeguard to your left should already be covering the zone and watching the rescue to see if you need help.)

Crossed Arms above the Head.   This signal stops dispatch and is generally used on slides, trollies, or other water attractions. It can be accompanied by one or two long whistle blasts indicating a rescue in progress. Two short whistle blasts to the dispatching lifeguard may indicate that the lifeguard at the bottom may need to retrieve a lost item for a guest (sunglasses, etc.) from the activity area or in the catch pool of a slide.

Thumbs Up.   Thumbs up resumes activity. It is usually accompanied by two short whistle blasts.

Tapping the Top of your Head. This signal means "watch my area" and is used with two short whistle blasts. It indicates that you would like your area watched momentarily. The lifeguard to your left should acknowledge and is then responsible for covering the area.

Other Communication Devices

In addition to whistle and hand signals, there are other communication devices that you need to be aware of.

Telephones. Telephones must be available for emergencies. The telephone numbers for emergency services must be posted at the telephone and clearly visible. It is also recommended that the number for the Poison Control Center be prominently displayed.

Cordless phones can be used, but a standard wall phone should also be available as a backup in case of malfunction of the cordless phone. If a pay telephone is the only means of communication available, and coins are needed to access emergency services, then the appropriate coin(s) should be taped in an available spot known only to employees. Hidden coins should be checked daily and replaced if missing. Emergency numbers should be displayed at such a telephone.

Larger waterparks and facilities have telephone systems to aid in lifeguard communication. They must be used only for official business and emergency purposes.

It is recommended that a verbal code be established to aid in quick communication of common information. If such a code is used in your facility, it will be explained in the EAS.

Walkie-Talkies. Walkie-talkies are used primarily for communication between supervisors and for the medical staff.

Public Address Systems. Loudspeaker systems are used for announcements, music, and other information of a general nature. If needed, emergency information can be communicated to your entire facility very quickly.

TEAM LIFEGUARDING

Once you activate the EAS, your signal draws together your lifeguard team. The team may be only you and the lifeguard to your left who covers your area and is ready to assist. If the situation is more serious, other lifeguards, your supervisor, and medical personnel may become part of your team.

Be aware that whatever the situation, there will always be someone to back you up. Remember also that you need to be prepared at all times to back up the lifeguard to your right.

All team members must know their parts in an emergency. This is why it is important to practice your EAS for a variety of emergency situ-

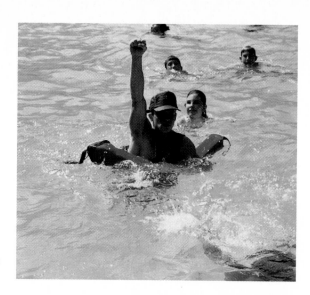

Know your part in an emergency.

ations. The ultimate goal is to successfully prevent drownings, and the more each staff member can be a part of the team process, the more effective your EAS will be.

RESCUES VS. ASSISTS

An **assist** occurs when you help a swimmer, either from on deck or in the water and are still able to maintain zone coverage within the 10/20 Protection Rule.

A **rescue** occurs when you must leave your post and cannot maintain the 10/20 Protection Rule within your zone while helping a distressed guest, or any situation in which the EAS is activated.

You always endanger your life and/or risk personal injury when you enter the water to rescue a guest.

RESCUE TUBES

Using a rescue tube for all rescues greatly reduces the danger and risk. In reviewing accident histories, it was discovered that traditional body contact rescues are not practical. They are **dangerous for the guest (victim) and dangerous for the lifeguard.**

The rescue tube has been proven to be the safest, most effective rescue device. All lifeguards must have a rescue tube at their post.

The techniques in this course are designed specifically for effective lifeguarding with the rescue tube.

The Rescue Tube on the Job

Special facilities lifeguards are required to wear their rescue tubes while on duty. Pool lifeguards, depending upon facility need and regulations, may wear their equipment or have it placed within arms' reach, where it is immediately available. Shallow water lifeguards also will wear or hold their equipment while lifeguarding.

To look professional and to have the rescue tube immediately available for assist and rescue use, you should wear the equipment in one of the following ways:

1. You may hold the tube in front of you.

2. You may hold it at your side while standing.

3. You may sit in the chair, with the rope secured in your hand and the tube across your lap.

In the following photos all lifeguards have rescue tubes, look professional, and can assist when necessary.

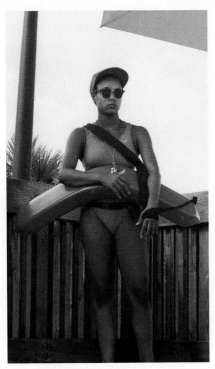 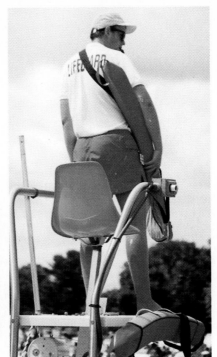 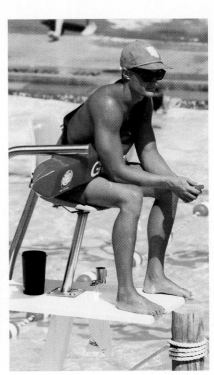

The rescue tube on the job.

REVIEW QUESTIONS

1. The Emergency Action System is activated by _____.

2. While a lifeguard is making a rescue, who covers the zone?

_____

3. Match the communication signal with its use:

_____	One short whistle	a. Major emergency
_____	Raised fist	b. Give direction
_____	Two long whistles	c. Gain swimmer attention
_____	Crossed arms	d. Watch my area
_____	Tapping head	e. Resume activity
_____	One long whistle	f. Rescue in progress
_____	Pointing	g. Lifeguard needs help
_____	Thumbs up	h. Stop dispatch

4. What should be posted next to the telephone?

   a.

   b.

   c.

5. What is the difference between an assist and a rescue? _____
   _____

6. Name three things you could use to make an extension assist.

   a.

   b.

   c.

7. When making an assist or a rescue, it is important to reassure the guest by _____ to him or her.

8. T   F   The rescue tube is an optional piece of equipment.

SKILL SHEET 2

Communications

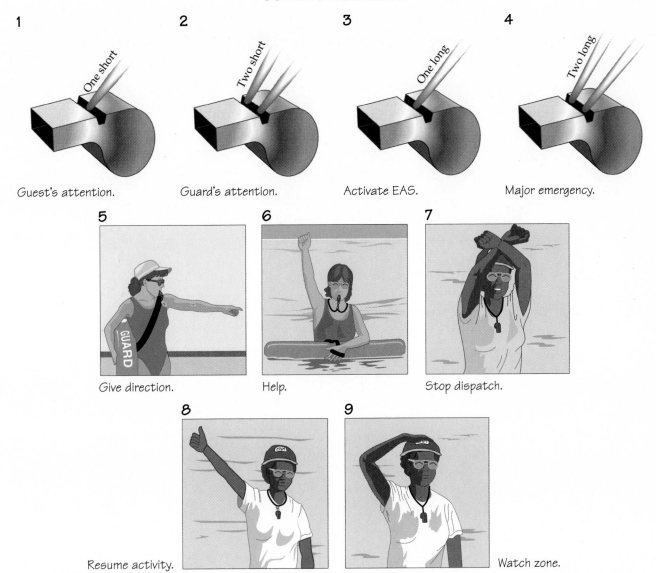

1
One short

Guest's attention.

2
Two short

Guard's attention.

3
One long

Activate EAS.

4
Two long

Major emergency.

5
Give direction.

6
Help.

7
Stop dispatch.

8
Resume activity.

9
Watch zone.

KEY POINTS:

◆ Blow whistle loudly and firmly.

◆ Combine whistle and hand signals.

◆ Avoid unnecessary communication; blow your whistle only when absolutely necessary.

CRITICAL THINKING:

1. What do you do if the guard to your right is making a rescue and raises a clenched fist?

2. When does an activity have to be cleared of remaining swimmers?

3. What is the difference between an assist and a rescue?

4. Why should a stand-mounted phone be used for emergency or business use only?

Management of a Distressed Guest on Top of the Water

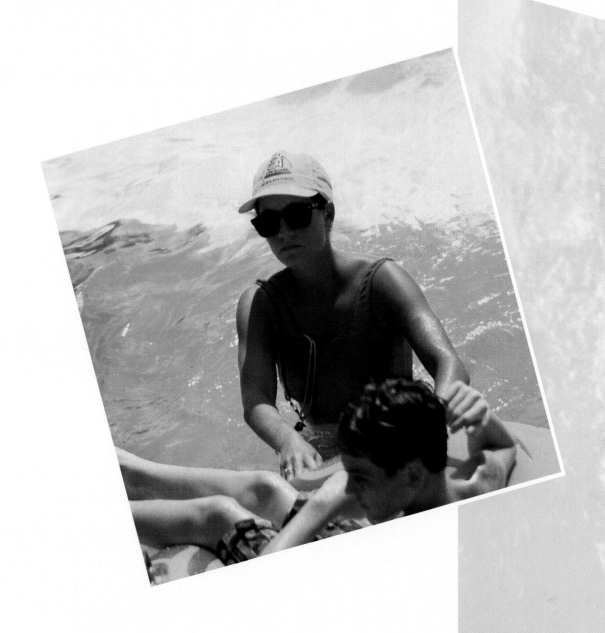

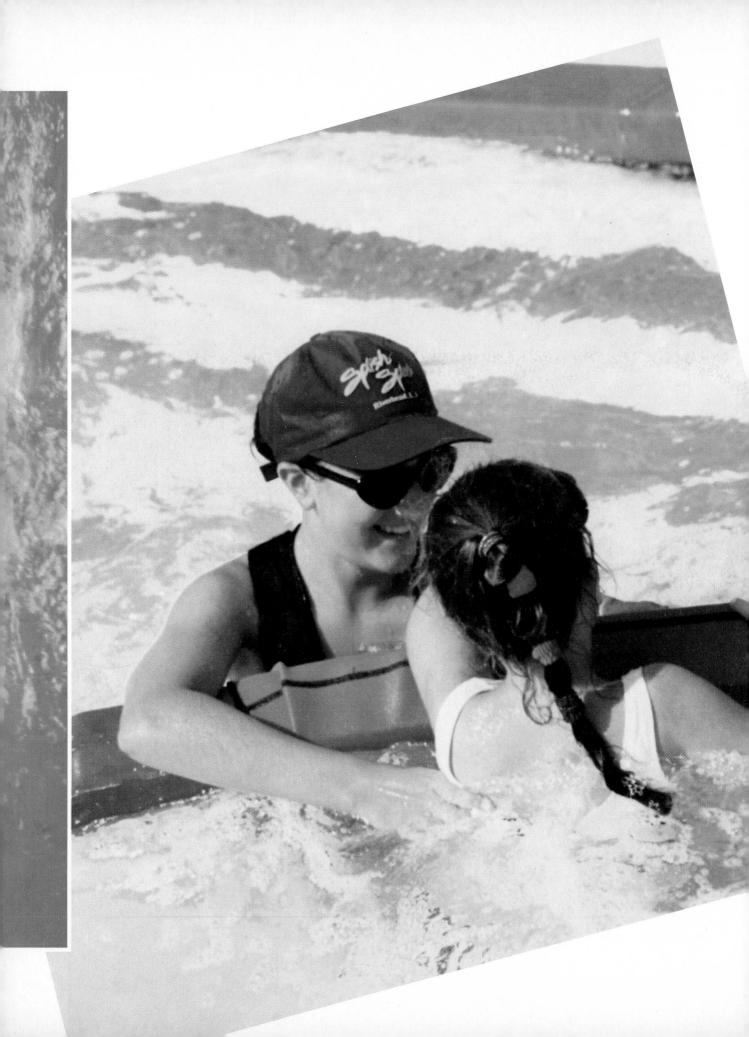

What Do I Need to Do If a Guest in Distress Is on Top of the Water and Still Breathing?

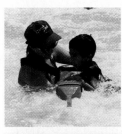

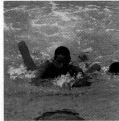

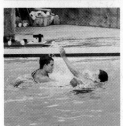

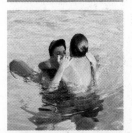

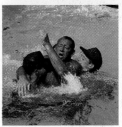

CHAPTER OBJECTIVES

After completing the chapter and related water work, the lifeguard candidate should be able to:

1. Identify the difference between a distressed swimmer and a near drowning.
2. Perform a compact jump entry and an approach stroke.
3. Perform a front drive.
4. Perform a rear huggie.
5. Integrate teamwork and front drive/rear huggie skills in a two-guard rescue.

Providing assistance to guests who need help can often be done without compromising your ability to maintain the 10/20 Protection Rule. As long as you can continue to maintain the 10/20 Protection Rule, any help you give is considered an **assist.** It is not necessary to activate your Emergency Action System or complete a rescue report for an assist.

ASSISTS

Guests may need an assist if they lose their footing, are slightly disoriented, have difficulty exiting the pool or standing up, or have a physical disability. You can assist these guests to safety by extending a body part, pole, rescue tube, or other device.

These types of assists are called reaching, or **extension assists,** and are usually done while standing, stooping, or lying on the pool deck. Or, if you are in the water (such as in a slide catch pool), you may also physically assist the guest, remembering to always keep your rescue tube between yourself and the individual you are assisting.

When executing an assist:

1. Provide reassurance by **talking to the guest** while doing the assist. You may be able to talk some guests to safety.

2. Remember that guests are generally able to assist themselves once they have grabbed an extension device.

3. After assisting the guest to safety, encourage measures to ensure the guest's safety for the remainder of the visit. This may include point

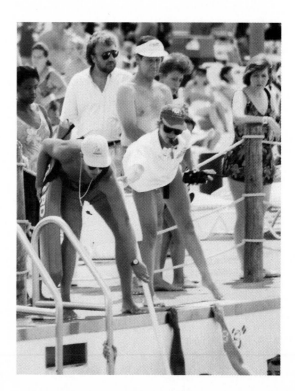

Extension assist.

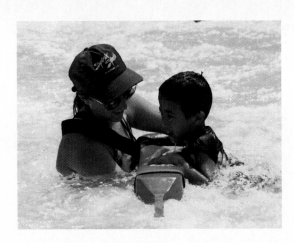
In-water assist.

ing out more appropriate areas of your facility for their ability level or suggesting use of a lifejacket or other risk management strategies. If you do suggest use of a lifejacket, remember that the buoyancy around the chest may make it difficult for some people to stand or regain their footing. You may need to continue to assist these guests until they get used to the lifejacket.

EXTENSION ASSISTS

Body Part

To use a body part for an extension assist:

1. Keep your body down low and your weight away from the water.

2. Grasp a stable part of the guest, such as the wrist or lower arm, rather than letting the guest grab you.

3. If you will need to assist a guest to the deck, grab underneath the guest's armpit as soon as possible to avoid shoulder injuries. Do **not** lift a person from the water by pulling on her arms.

4. Once a guest is pulled to safety and she wants to get out of the water, assist until the guest is out of the pool.

Pole Extension

To use a pole extension for an extension assist:

1. Keep your body weight as low to the deck as possible and lean back away from the water's edge.

2. Extend the pole out slightly beyond and to the side of the guest.

3. Slowly bring the pole toward the guest. Encourage the guest to reach for and grab the pole. A distressed nonswimmer may have his eyes closed, or hair and water may be blocking the guest's vision. Touch the extension device against the guest's arm or shoulder.

4. When the guest has grasped the pole, pull him to the side by slowly sweeping the pole toward the edge of the pool.

5. Be cautious of other guests in the water and of those who may be standing behind you.

Rescue Tube or Other Extension Device

To use a rescue tube or other extension device for an extension assist:

1. When you use equipment in an assist, the guest may be unable to see the device even when it is within reach. You may need to place the equipment in the person's hands.

2. It is important that the equipment be within the guest's reach, but you must be careful not to hit the guest with the equipment.

3. Once the guest is holding onto the equipment, bring her to the side of the pool and assist her out of the water if she wishes to exit the area.

4. Assists can be done in either shallow or deep water. You must make the judgment of whether or not you can continue to maintain the 10/20 Protection Rule while assisting the guest. If not, activate your Emergency Action System by blowing one long whistle blast, and execute a **rescue.**

RESCUES

A rescue is any situation that requires you to enter the water and help a guest in distress, which would prevent you from continuing to maintain the 10/20 Protection Rule in your zone. You must activate your Emergency Action System by blowing one long whistle blast before you enter the water. A rescue report must also be completed after the rescue has been accomplished. For documentation and reporting purposes, rescues will be classified in two ways, depending upon the severity of the incident.

DISTRESSED SWIMMER VS. NEAR DROWNING RESCUE

A **distressed swimmer rescue** involves a guest who exhibited behavior indicating an inability to remain upon, or return to, the surface of the water. The situation would have resulted in death by drowning if the swimmer was not aided by a lifeguard. In all such cases, the distressed swimmer is rescued by a lifeguard before the situation becomes life threatening.

A **near drowning rescue** involves an individual who is rendered unconscious during an immersion incident, rescued by the lifeguard, and successfully revived by the initiation of CPR and advanced life support Emergency Medical Services. In all such cases, the victims of a near drowning incident recover and survive the episode.

ENTRY AND APPROACH

The first step in making an effective rescue is entering the water in an efficient and safe way. The **compact jump entry** is used to enter the water to do a rescue. It is always accompanied by one long whistle blast to activate your Emergency Action System, and it is done with the rescue tube. You must keep your eyes on the victim while preparing to jump:

1. Put the rescue tube strap on diagonally across your chest.

2. Gather the rope in some manner so that it will not hook onto anything as you jump. The rope can be held in your hand, tied in a slip knot, or secured by any manner that keeps it out of the way, yet will allow full extension of the strap after your entry.

3. Bring the rescue tube up across your chest, reach over the tube with both arms, and press it toward your body to lock it into place.

4. Jump from the lifeguard chair or pool deck, keeping your legs together. **Do not point your toes. Keep your feet flat.** If you hit the bottom with pointed toes, you could break them!

5. As you reach the water, bend your knees as if you are sitting in a chair and be prepared to hit the bottom with **flat feet.**

6. You may go underneath the water briefly, but you will surface quickly because of the buoyancy of the rescue tube.

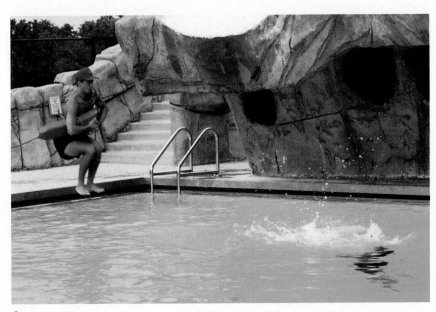

Compact jump.

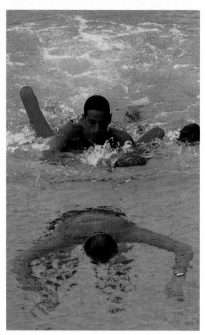

Approach stroke.

After entering the water with a compact jump entry, you need to get to the distressed guest as quickly as possible. Your **approach stroke** can be any combination of leg kicks and arm movements that allows you to make the fastest forward progress in the water. The most effective kick for most lifeguards will be either the breaststroke kick or the flutter kick, combined with either the breaststroke or crawl arm stroke.

When you are approach stroking:

1. Keep the rescue tube in front of your chest, **between you and the distressed guest at all times.** Do not pull it behind you. Keeping the tube in front of you allows you to be in the best position to do the rescue and reduces the chance of other guests grabbing the equipment. (The only exception to this would be if there is an area of your facility that compromises the 10/20 Protection Rule if a tube is used during **initial** approach stroking, and it is more effective to have the tube in another position. For example, if you had to swim through a current or out from some lakefronts. In these cases, **upon the granting of a variance by** Ellis & Associates, the tube could be pulled behind during approach stroking until you are approximately 3 body lengths (15–20 feet) from the distressed guest. At that point, the tube should be pulled into the approach stroke position.)

2. Keep your eyes on the distressed guest at all times.

3. The rescue tube strap may be worn across your chest or held along with the equipment.

FRONT DRIVE AND REAR HUGGIE

As you approach stroke toward the distressed guest on the surface of the water, he will be either facing toward you (so you will execute a **front drive**) or facing away from you (so you will execute a **rear huggie**). These rescue skills can be done in either shallow or deep water.

Front Drive

To execute a front drive:

1. Whistle, push the E-stop button if you are working at a wave pool, do a compact jump entry, and approach stroke toward the distressed guest.

2. When you are about 6–10 feet from the guest, pull the rescue tube from underneath your arms, and push it out in front of you with both hands. Keep your arms straight with your elbows locked. Keep the tube pushed out in front of you as far as possible.

3. As you near the guest, use your strongest kick to push the tube slightly underwater and into the chest of the distressed guest, "driving" the guest backward. The rescue tube should be in such a position that the guests' arms are over it.

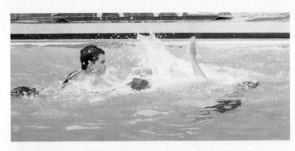

Push the tube out in front of you.

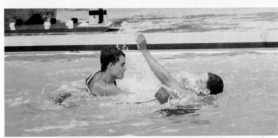

Drive the tube into the guest's chest.

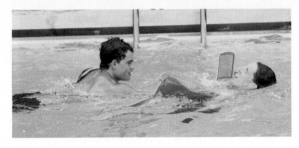

Keep driving.

4. **Keep kicking and driving,** moving the guest backward while maintaining your momentum. Tell the guest you are a lifeguard and are there to help. Encourage the guest to hold onto the rescue tube. Try to stay on your stomach with your hips up toward the surface of the water.

5. Make progress toward an exit point or the side of the pool. Keep your elbows straight and arms locked. **Continue to talk** to the guest for reassurance. You can even ask the guest to help you kick toward the side.

6. Secure the guest at the side of the pool, assist the guest from the water, and fill out the rescue report.

If for some reason the guest grabs you during a front drive rescue, there are several things you can do to prevent injury to yourself while still maintaining an effective rescue:

1. Use a front huggie position. **As long as you have the rescue tube between yourself and the guest** and both of your heads are above water, you can still continue to safely make progress toward an exit or side of the pool. After the distressed guest grabs you, reach under the guest's arms and "hug." It is very important for you to keep your head and body a little to the side of the distressed guest so he cannot

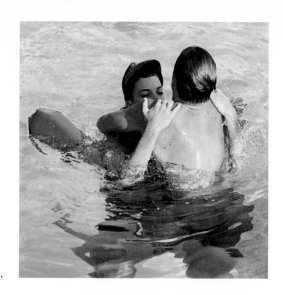

The front huggie.

hurt you if his head moves sharply while you are in the front huggie position.

2. If you find yourself being pushed underwater, execute a flip-over so that you are on top of the guest moving forward, and the guest is on his back. Keep kicking and use the guest's effort to help leverage the flip. Try not to allow yourself to be forced into a vertical position or on your back. **Keep the rescue tube between you and the guest.**

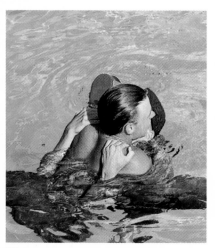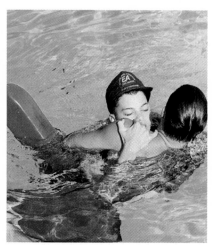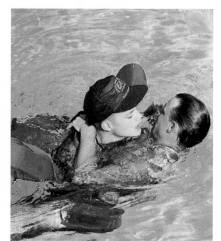

Flip-over.

3. If the guest has grabbed you in such a way that you cannot continue the rescue, get some air, tuck your head, and submerge. Push yourself away from the guest, recover your tube so that it is between you and the distressed guest, and either reapproach or signal for help from a second lifeguard.

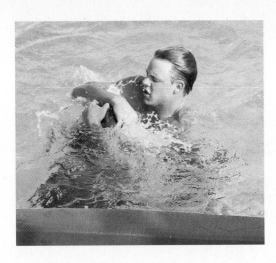

Push away.

Rear Huggie

To execute a rear huggie:

1. Whistle, push the E-stop button if you are working at a wave pool, and approach to a position directly behind the distressed guest.

2. Keep the tube in your approach stroke position, right up against your chest, under your armpits.

3. Watch the distressed guest's movements, and as quickly as possible, extend your arms under the guest's armpits and wrap them around her chest. This can be done even if the guest is slightly underwater.

4. Keep your body a little to the side of the guest, with your head turned to the side to avoid injury if the guest suddenly snaps her head back sharply.

5. Immediately begin talking to the guest, being sure that the rescue tube remains between the two of you.

6. Proceed toward an exit point or side of the pool, secure the guest and assist her from the water, and fill out the rescue report.

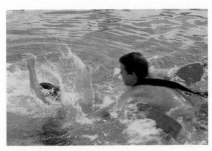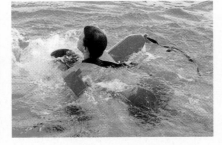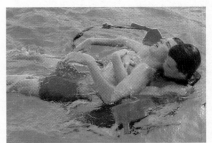

The rear huggie.

TWO-GUARD RESCUE

Occasionally, a distressed guest on the surface may be too active for one lifeguard to handle. This is especially true if the guest is under the influence of alcohol or drugs. A two-guard rescue combines both the front drive and rear huggie into a "sandwich" that can control even the most difficult guests.

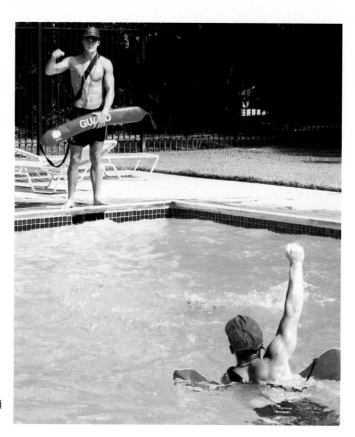

Two-guard rescue.

If you feel you need assistance while making a rescue:

1. Raise your fist above your head, while continuing to attempt the rescue by driving forward and **talking to the distressed guest.** Keep your hips up and stay horizontal for your own protection.

2. At this point, the secondary lifeguard (the one whose station is to the **left** of yours) whistles.

3. **The remaining lifeguards clear the pool while covering the open zones.**

4. The secondary lifeguard does a compact jump entry and approach strokes to a position on the other side of the distressed guest, opposite you. You should still be attempting to drive, keeping your hips up. The secondary rescuer should also keep his hips as high as possible.

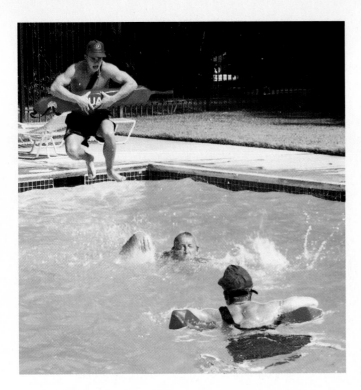

Two-guard
rescue.

5. At this point, the lifeguard who is behind the distressed guest will prepare to do a **rear huggie.** When possible, it is helpful if the lifeguards communicate with each other so that the lifeguard in front knows when the rear lifeguard will begin the rear huggie and thus can prepare for the front drive. It does not matter which lifeguard does which skill; it depends on the position of the distressed guest.

6. The lifeguard doing the rear huggie should bring his forearms up to present a "target" for the front drive.

7. The front lifeguard then front drives into the distressed guest, aiming for the target presented by the rear lifeguard. As soon as the res

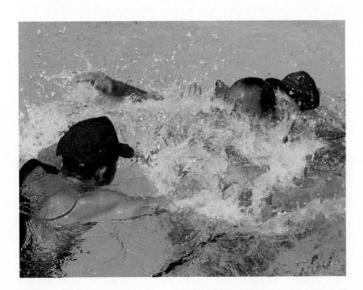

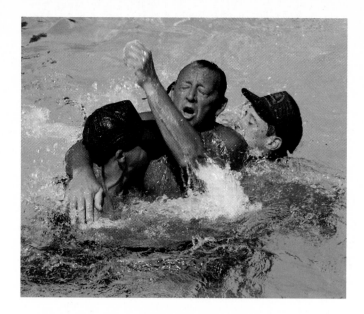

cue tube contacts the arms of the rear lifeguard, this lifeguard should reach **over** the rescue tube to secure it and lock in the guest.

8. The rear huggie and front drive should be done as close to the same time as possible. Communication is helpful so that both lifeguards are ready to execute their rescue about the same time.

9. While watching the distressed guest and the rear lifeguard, the front lifeguard starts to push or tow the pair to an exit area. The lifeguards should continue to talk to the guest to reassure them while kicking toward safety.

10. Secure the guest, assist the guest out of the water, and complete the rescue report.

REVIEW QUESTIONS

1. T   F   The difference between a **distressed swimmer rescue** and a **near drowning rescue** is that in a near drowning the guest is unconscious and successfully revived by the lifeguard, and a distressed swimmer is rescued before the situation becomes life-threatening.

2. T   F   The compact jump entry is performed with the legs apart.

3. T   F   In order for a front drive to be successful, you must keep your arms straight and keep driving by kicking as hard as you can.

4. T   F   Active guests in distress can be approached from the front or the rear.

5. T   F   Communication between lifeguards in a two-guard rescue is not important.

6. Why is it important to always try to grab underneath the armpit, as soon as possible, when assisting a victim?

SKILL SHEET 3

The Front Drive

1

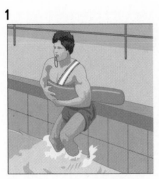

Whistle; compact jump with feet flat.

2

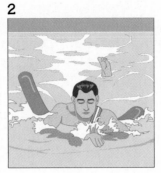

Approach stroke; kick and pull.

3

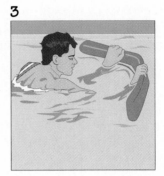

Extend tube; lock elbows.

4

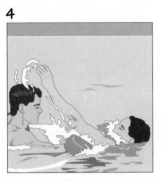

Drive tube; keep kicking.

5

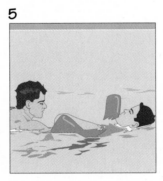

Keep driving; talk.

6

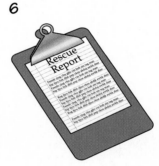

Secure guest at side; complete rescue report.

KEY POINTS:

◆ Keep kicking—hips up!

◆ Push tube slightly underwater before driving.

◆ Get tube under guest's arms.

◆ Keep talking; have guest hold onto tube.

◆ Keep tube between yourself and the guest.

CRITICAL THINKING:

1. What are some of the things you can do if a guest grabs you while you are executing a front drive?

2. Why should you talk to the guest? What should you say?

3. What type of distressed guest is the front drive rescue designed for?

SKILL SHEET 4

Rear Huggie

CONSCIOUS GUEST:

1
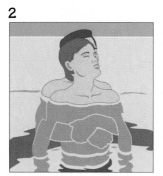
Whistle; compact jump; approach stroke.

2
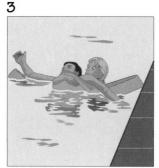
Hug under armpits, around body.

3
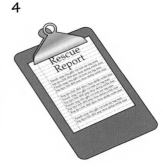
Talk; proceed to side.

4

Secure and remove; complete rescue report.

UNCONSCIOUS GUEST:

1
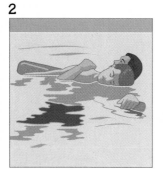
Whistle; compact jump; approach stroke.

2
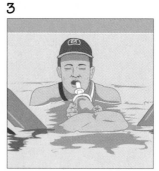
Hug around body, pull back onto tube.

3
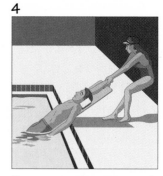
Give rescue breathing with pocket mask according to protocol.

4

Extricate and continue with rescue breathing/CPR protocol.

KEY POINTS:

- Keep your body off-center and your head down.
- Kick—keep moving after contact.
- Keep tube next to your body, under your armpits.

CRITICAL THINKING:

1. What could you do if the guest suddenly became unconscious during your rescue after you had completed the rear huggie?
2. What would you do if the guest struggles?
3. What would you do if the guest slips off the tube?
4. What if the guest is too big for you to wrap your arms around?

SKILL SHEET 5

Two-Guard Rescue

1

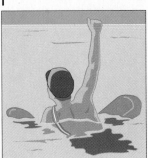

Signal for help; keep trying to drive.

2

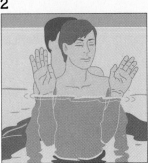

Guard behind does rear huggie—"target."

3

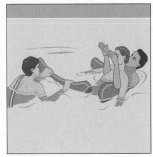

Guard in front does front drive.

4

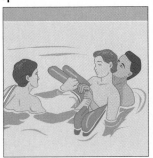

Rear guard locks hands over front tube.

5

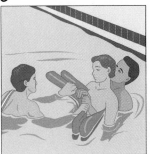

Talk to guest; progress to side.

6

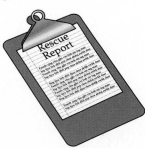

Secure and remove guest; complete rescue report.

KEY POINTS:

◆ Keep hips up.

◆ Communicate.

◆ Rear huggie and front drive at same time if possible.

◆ Watch your head—keep it down.

◆ Practice being first and second rescuer.

CRITICAL THINKING:

1. What would you do if the guest became unconscious after the rescue was completed?

2. What is necessary for effective teamwork?

3. What situations might cause a guest to be out of control and make a two-guard rescue necessary?

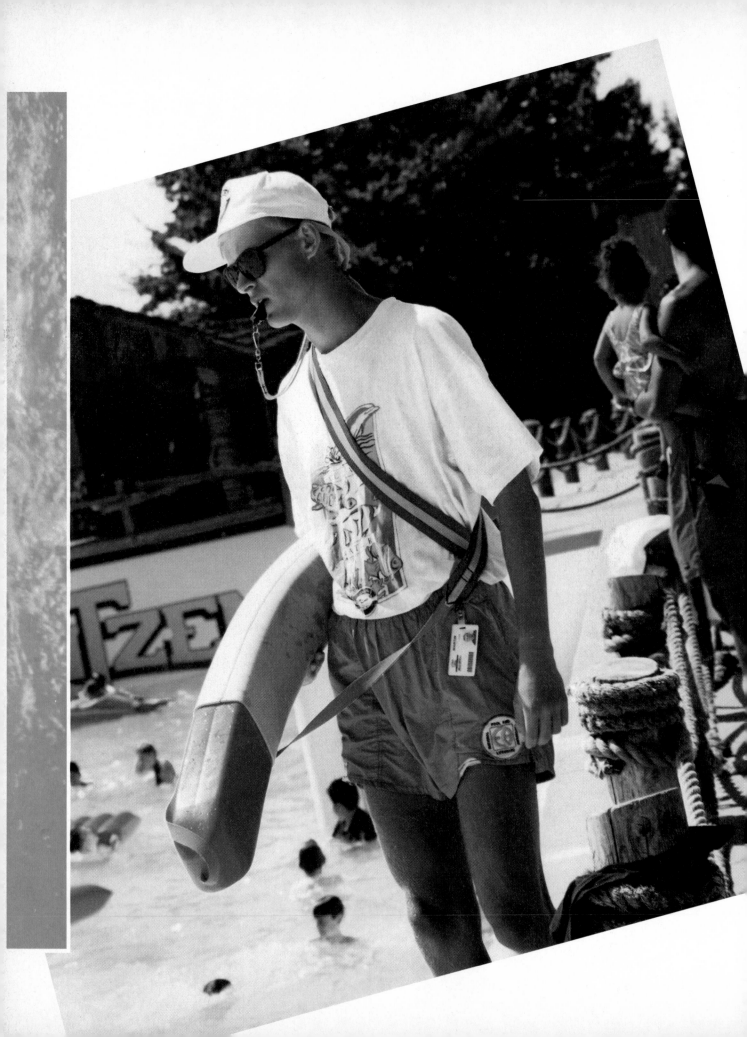

What Do I Do If a Guest in Distress Is on Top of the Water and Is Not Breathing?

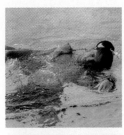

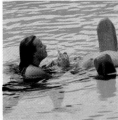

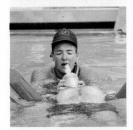

CHAPTER OBJECTIVES

After completing the chapter and related water work, the lifeguard candidate should be able to:

1. Adapt the rear huggie to an unconscious guest.
2. Understand the importance of rescue breathing in the water.
3. Understand the importance of Universal Precautions.
4. Open the airway, place a pocket mask, and rescue breathe in the water.
5. Quickly and safely remove an unconscious guest from the water.

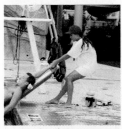

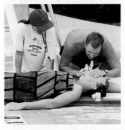

49

I f a guest is unconscious in the water, he may be floating face down on the surface. An unconscious guest needs to be quickly turned over and placed on a rescue tube so that you can begin rescue breathing immediately. Those first few seconds and minutes are critical for the successful outcome of the emergency.

REAR HUGGIE—UNCONSCIOUS GUEST

A rear huggie is the most effective method of getting an unconscious guest on the rescue tube and in a position to maintain an open airway. It is performed the same way as for an active guest on the surface, with the following modifications:

1. Swim to a position behind the guest if you need to. You will have to be almost on top of the guest to get your arms under his armpits and wrapped around the chest.

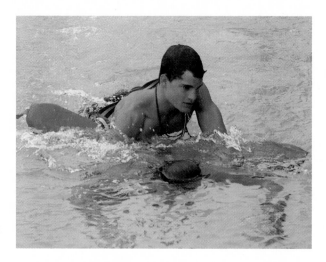

Wrap arms around guest.

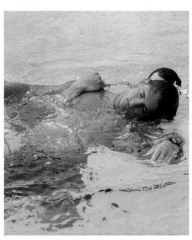

Kick and pull guest back onto rescue tube.

2. Pull the guest backwards so that he is face up, with the tube under the upper back. Kick your legs to help as you pull. You can also roll the guest to get him into the face up position. Use the method that works best for you. Remember to watch out for the guest's head as you pull him back or roll him over.

3. Be sure the tube is under the guest's back. Move to a position at the top of the guest's head. An unconscious guest's head will naturally fall back into an open airway position if the tube is properly placed under the back.

Make sure the guest's airway is open. The tongue of an unconscious person usually collapses against the back of the throat and interferes with oxygen reaching the lungs. Tilting the head back will unblock the throat and allow an open air passage. Look at the position that an unconscious guest will be in when placed on the rescue tube correctly. This is an ideal open airway position.

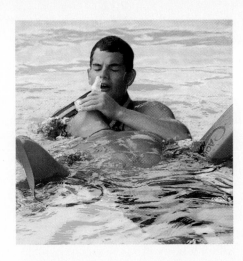

Immediately begin rescue breathing with pocket mask.

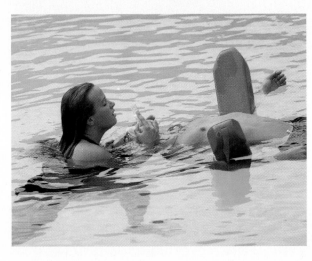

Open airway position on rescue tube.

If the guest is breathing, continue making progress to the side, remove the guest from the water, and continue your assessment according to your Lifeguard First Responder protocols.

If the guest is not breathing, you will need to begin rescue breathing **immediately.**

RESCUE BREATHING IN THE WATER

Lack of air to the brain can rapidly lead to irreversible brain damage. That is why it is so important to begin rescue breathing as quickly as possible. In most cases, it will take you more than 1 minute to get a guest to the side and out of the pool. That first minute is critical.

Also of critical importance is protection from the possible transmission of disease if you should come in contact with a guest's body fluids while giving rescue breathing. While administering breaths to a non-breathing guest in the water, you will use a protective mask that is designed to form an effective "seal" in the water. You must become very familiar with the specific masks that are used by your facility. Practice is the only acceptable method for maintaining a high level of skill in using the mask in the water for rescue breathing.

UNIVERSAL PRECAUTIONS

Always using the mask when performing rescue breathing in the water is part of an aggressive, standardized approach to infection control known as Universal Precautions. According to this concept, you should treat all human blood and body fluids as if they are known to contain human immunodeficiency virus (causes AIDS) or hepatitis B virus or other blood-borne diseases. There is no way for you to know in advance if you will or will not come in contact with body fluids or if they will be contaminated. Therefore, in any situation in which there is the possibility of exposure, you must use some type of barrier to protect you. When you are performing rescue breathing or CPR, you will use the mask. If there is bleeding present, you will need to use latex gloves. Your facility will give you more detailed and specific training in blood-borne pathogens, exposure control, and Universal Precautions to let you know what they will provide for your protection while you are on the job.

USE OF THE MASK IN THE WATER

After you have determined that the guest is not breathing, call out the fact that you have a nonbreathing guest to your backup lifeguards so that they can follow up according to your facility Emergency Action Plan (EAP). In some facilities, every lifeguard may enter the water with a mask. At others, the mask may be brought to you by your backup lifeguard. Common sense, enforcement of the 10/20 Protection Rule, and your facility Emergency Action Plan will determine how and when this mask will be used. To begin rescue breathing in the water with the mask:

1. Open the airway by placing the guest on the rescue tube. The guest's mouth should be open, but protect it from going underwater or from water splashing in.

2. Shake out any water from the valve of the mask.

3. Place the mask over the guest's nose and mouth. Make sure that the valve is directly over the guest's mouth.

4. Wrap your hand and fingers around the mask in such a way that you can apply even, firm pressure to keep the mask in place and make the seal. You will need to practice this skill with the masks that your facility uses, as each mask is shaped differently.

5. Get up close to the guest so that you can put your mouth on the valve. If you need to, use the end of the rescue tube for support to get your body high enough to reach the valve. Depending upon the mask

you use, a position at the top of the head, looking toward the guest's feet, may be the most efficient.

6. Take a full, deep breath, wrap your lips around the valve, and exhale strongly. Give a second breath. If the air does not go into the guest (try putting your mask against your arm and exhaling into the valve; this is what a blocked airway will feel like), re-tilt the guest's head, and try again. If air still does not go in, proceed to the side, extricate the guest quickly, and use the treatment for an obstructed airway.

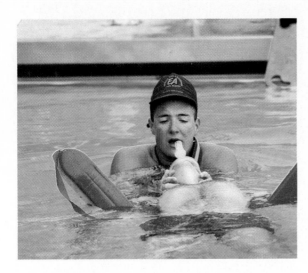

Rescue breathing with mask in the water.

7. After the initial 2 breaths, breath at a rate of 1 breath every 5 seconds (for an adult). Count 1 one-thousand, 2 one-thousand, 3 one-thousand, 4 one-thousand, **breathe.** Count **out loud** and confidently when you practice. This will help make the skills of rescue breathing in the water easier to perform under the pressure of a real emergency because you will be used to performing in a specific way that will become automatic if you **practice consistently.**

8. Continue making progress to the side of the pool and prepare to quickly extricate the guest from the pool, where you will assess the guest's airway, breathing, and circulation.

EXTRICATION

Removing an unconscious guest from the pool to the deck by lifting, or "popping-up," can be difficult and cause injury to either you or the guest. This is especially true if the guest is large. By using a backboard (which is a required piece of equipment at each facility), an unconscious guest can be removed from the pool quickly and safely. This technique is used only when the guest is unconscious and you **do not suspect a spinal injury.** As with the other rescue techniques, you will need to practice this skill at your facility and with your equipment so that you are familiar with the locations of your backboards and how the board performs. Each area of your facility may have different water/deck levels or types of ledges or gutters that may affect the execution of this technique. To remove an unconscious guest who does not have a spinal injury:

1. The rescuing lifeguard assesses the guest, calls out findings or calls for the board, and begins rescue breathing while making progress to the side of the pool.

2. The second lifeguard brings the backboard, removes the head immobilizer, and places the backboard in the water (straight up and down) against the pool wall.

3. As the rescuing lifeguard brings the guest to the board, the second lifeguard stabilizes the board with one hand while grabbing the upper arm of the guest with the other and **maintaining this contact.**

4. The rescuing lifeguard slides the rescue tube from under the guest, being sure to slide it out before the guest makes contact with the board. If the water is deep, the rescuing lifeguard can use the tube for her own support. The guest should be quickly straightened on the board and moved to the end of the backboard.

5. The second lifeguard will now **pull,** while the first lifeguard **pushes** the board out of the water and onto the deck. The lifeguards must coordinate with each other so they both pull and push together. The "see-saw" effect created when the board is pushed up along the edge of the gutter allows the board and guest to come onto the deck easily. The removal of the guest from the pool using the backboard should be **quick** and **efficient.** If a guest is extremely large or the pool deck is very high from the water surface, a body strap, placed high up under the guest's arm pits may be needed.

6. The lifeguards move the board to a level area and continue rescue breathing. The guest's pulse should be assessed and the appropriate protocols followed while awaiting arrival of the Emergency Medical Services.

If you have signaled for help and a backup guard is in the water with you, the extrication with the backboard could be quickly performed using three lifeguards:

Use of backboard for nonspinal removal from the water.

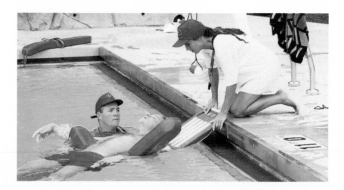

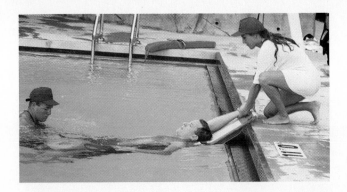

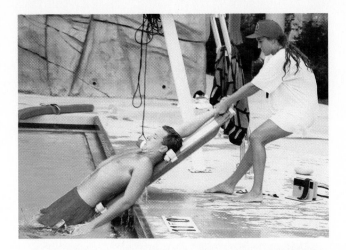

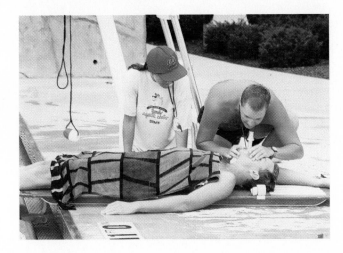

1. The second lifeguard enters the water with the pocket mask (if the rescuing lifeguard does not have it) and begins rescue breathing. The third lifeguard gets the backboard.

2. As the first and second lifeguards approach the wall, the second lifeguard moves to the guest's side opposite the first lifeguard and continues rescue breathing.

3. The first lifeguard (rescuing lifeguard) removes the rescue tube from under the guest's back and places it under his own armpits. He holds

the guest, and with the other hand, gives the guest's arm to the third lifeguard on deck.

4. As the third lifeguard elevates the backboard under the guest, the first lifeguard removes his arm.

5. The second lifeguard gives the last breath before removal. The third lifeguard pulls on the board and holds the guest's arm. The first lifeguard pushes the board on to the deck. While the board is being removed from the pool, the second lifeguard hops on the deck to assist in the removal, and then continues rescue breathing for one breath. The guest's pulse is then checked, and proper protocols are followed for continued care.

REVIEW QUESTIONS

1. List three things you may have to do to adapt a rear huggie for use with an unconscious guest.

   a.

   b.

   c.

2. Why is it important to start rescue breathing in the water?

3. T F   Universal Precautions means to treat **all** body fluids as if they are contaminated and take measures to protect yourself from exposure to them.

4. T F   Placing an unconscious guest on the rescue tube, with the tube under the back, is usually an ideal open airway position.

5. Four reasons for using a pocket mask in the water are:

   a.

   b.

   c.

   d.

6. T F   When removing an unconscious guest from the water, it is important to do it quickly and with minimal risk of injury to the guest or to you.

7. The rate of rescue breathing in the water for an adult is one breath every _____ seconds.

8. The rate of rescue breathing in the water for a child is one breath every _____ seconds.

9. T F   Another word for removal is **extrication.**

10. T F   A method of removing an unconscious nonspinal injured guest that is both quick and safe is to use a backboard, without the straps or head piece, using the two-lifeguard technique.

SKILL SHEET 6

Nonspinal Extrication

1

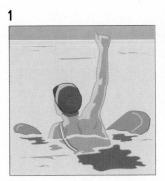

Signal for help.

2

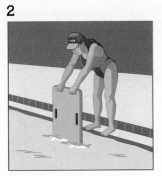

Proceed to side; place backboard (second lifeguard); continues rescue breathing (first lifeguard).

3

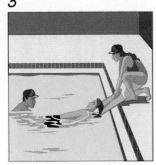

Remove tube and place guest (first lifeguard); place guest and grab arm (second lifeguard).

4

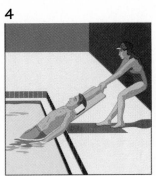

Maintain contact with arm and pull board on deck (second lifeguard); push board on deck (first lifeguard).

5

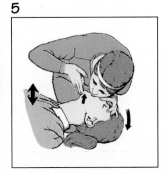

Continue with proper rescue breathing/CPR protocols.

KEY POINTS:	CRITICAL THINKING:

KEY POINTS:

- ◆ Perform quickly!
- ◆ Communicate.
- ◆ Maintain contact with guest.
- ◆ Careful removal of the backboard.
- ◆ Use the backboard and side of pool as a fulcrum.

CRITICAL THINKING:

1. When would this skill be used?
2. What if for some reason your backboard was not readily available, and it would take a minute or so for it to arrive? What are your options?

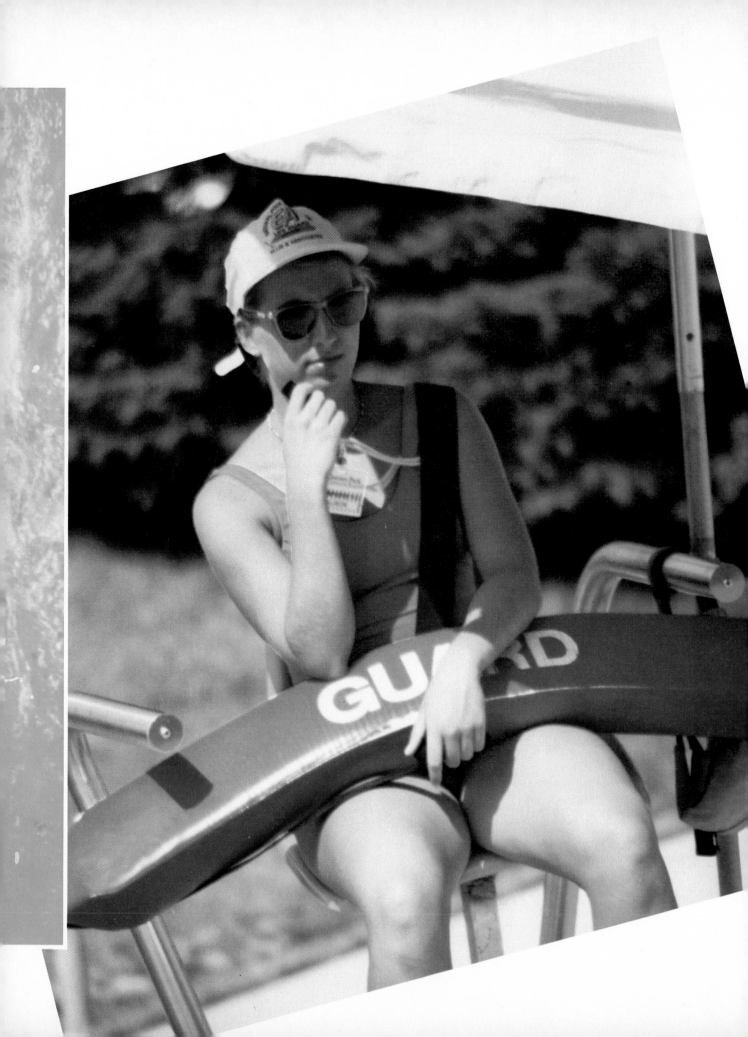

What Do I Do If a Guest Loses His Pulse?

5

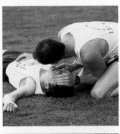

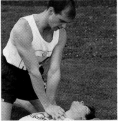

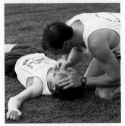

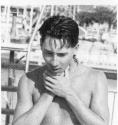

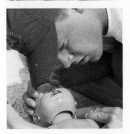

CHAPTER OBJECTIVES

After completing the chapter and related water work, the lifeguard candidate should be able to:

1. Understand the concept of CPR.
2. Conduct a primary survey.
3. Perform proper chest compression techniques for adult, child, and infant.
4. Know the ratios for breaths to compressions for adult, child, and infant.
5. Remove a foreign body airway obstruction from an adult, child, or infant, conscious or unconscious.
6. Perform two-lifeguard CPR.

For several years, lifeguards have been saving countless lives using a basic resuscitation technique called cardiopulmonary resuscitation or CPR. Components of this technique include assessing unresponsiveness, activating the Emergency Action Services (EAS)/Emergency Medical Services (EMS), opening the airway, assessing breathing, and performing rescue breathing (artificial ventilations), pulse check, and chest compressions. As lifeguard first responders, you will become proficient in the skills of assessing the patient's level of consciousness, activating the EAS/EMS, and completing a primary survey. Review these important skills often!

This chapter will focus on those specific life-saving skills that are critical for the pulseless and/or nonbreathing patient. CPR skills related to the adult patient are presented first. Techniques in CPR for children are then presented. Finally, attention will center on the CPR techniques for infants. In each of the sections, information on foreign body airway obstruction management is simultaneously covered. Contrary to many professional opinions, CPR skills are easy to learn and if practiced often, easy to recall. The lifeguard first responder should always remember that by recognizing an emergency situation and taking the appropriate **action,** the injured guest's chances for a positive outcome are drastically improved.

CARDIOPULMONARY DEFINITIONS

"Cardio" refers to the heart and "pulmonary" refers to the lungs. Therefore, cardiopulmonary resuscitation (CPR) is a set of assessment techniques and "hands on" skills that attempt to assist the heart and lungs to function after they have stopped and until advanced cardiac life support can be provided.

CPR and Blood-Borne Pathogens

The lifeguard first responder should use appropriate barriers when involved in any emergency situation. During resuscitation events, injured guests commonly vomit and expose the lifeguard first responder to body fluids. At a minimum, a mouth-to-barrier device should be used.

CARDIOPULMONARY RESUSCITATION TECHNIQUES (ADULT)

Just like any other emergency situation, the lifeguard first responder should first complete a scene survey to ensure rescuer safety. Immediately after this survey, begin the primary survey.

Steps in the Primary Survey

1. Determine the level of consciousness (shake the guest and shout, "Are you OK?").

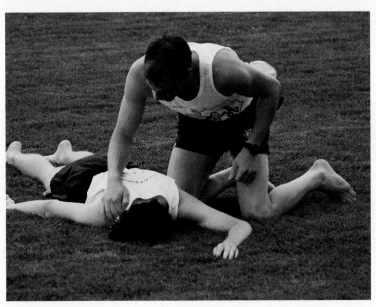

Shake and shout.

2. If the guest does not respond and appears unconscious, immediately activate the EAS/EMS. If the injured guest is lying on his or her stomach, gently roll the guest onto the back. If you suspect neck injury, request assistance and logroll the guest onto the back. Attempt to maintain an imaginary straight line between the nose and naval while logrolling the body as a unit.

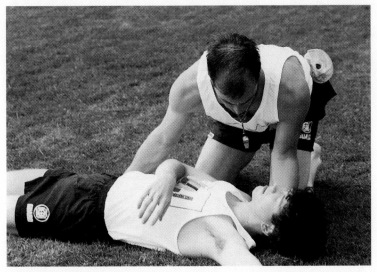

Roll injured guest onto back, protecting head.

3. Open the guest's airway (A = airway) using the head-tilt, chin-lift method or in the case of a suspected head or neck injury, the jaw thrust.

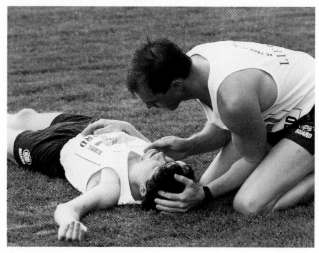

Open airway.

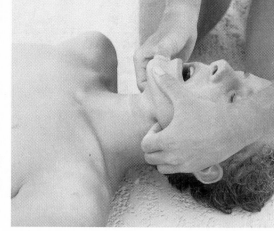

Jaw thrust.

4. Determine the status of breathing (B = breathing) by looking at the chest for movement, listening for air passing through the nose and mouth, and feeling for exhaled air against your cheek.

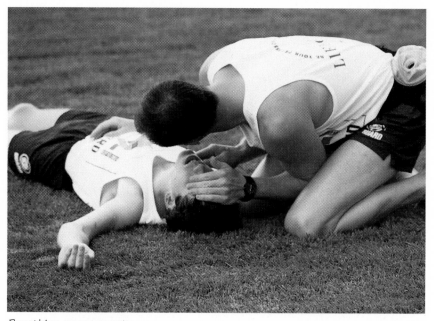

Breathing assessment.

5. If the guest is breathing, he or she also has a pulse (C = pulse). If you do not suspect any neck or back injury, place the guest in the recovery position and continue to monitor the ABC's.

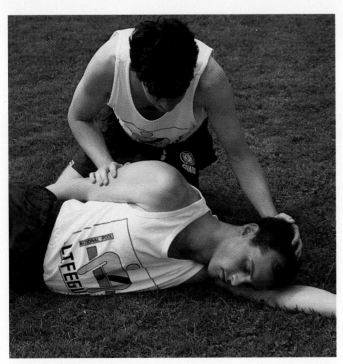

Recovery position.

6. If the guest is not breathing seal the airway barrier over the mouth and nose and give two full breaths. If you don't have a barrier that covers the nose, you must pinch the nose shut. Each breath should be slow, taking 1-1/2 to 2 seconds including (inhalation and exhalation) to complete. Watch the rise and fall of the chest during each breath.

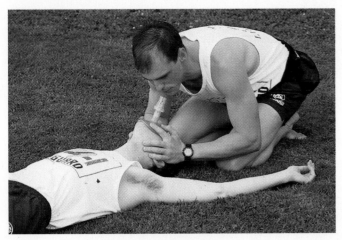

Mouth-to-mouth breathing with mask.

If you are unable to create a good seal around the mouth, consider mouth-to-nose breaths. This also is the method of choice for injured guests with oral trauma or clinched teeth.

7. If the initial breath is unsuccessful, reposition the injured guest's airway and then attempt two more breaths. If these are also unsuccessful, immediately begin foreign body airway obstruction (choking) removal techniques.

8. Once you have successfully given the guest two breaths, assess the pulse.

9. An adult's pulse is assessed at a carotid artery found in the neck. Using two or three fingers, find the Adam's apple and slide your fingers into the groove on the side closest to you. Take between 5 and 10 seconds to assess the pulse.

Stop Reading! Try and find your own carotid pulse before continuing. Count the number of beats in 15 seconds and multiply this number by 4. Example: 20 beats (in 15 seconds) multiplied by 4 = 80 beats per minute.

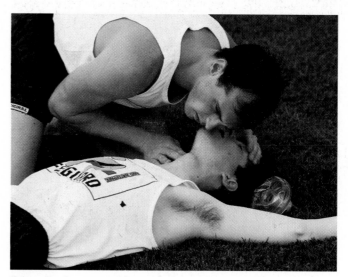

Pulse check at carotid arteries.

10. If the guest has a pulse and is not breathing, begin rescue breathing techniques and continuously monitor the pulse.

11. If no pulse can be found, you must begin CPR by alternating chest compressions and rescue breathing.

CHEST COMPRESSION TECHNIQUES (ADULT)

In order to perform chest compressions properly, the lifeguard first responder must find the correct hand position or landmark. Placing your hands in any other position places the injured guest at higher risk for serious additional injuries, (i.e., collapsed lungs, lacerated abdominal organs including the liver, stomach, and intestine):

1. To find the correct chest compression landmark, the guest's clothing should either be ripped away or pushed up around the shoulders.

(Maintain the guest's modesty if possible.) Kneel aside the guest's chest and run your fingers up along the rib cage as shown. Find the end of the breastbone where the two sides of the rib cage meet. A notch can be felt.

2. Place your middle finger on the notch and index finger next to it.

   Stop Reading! Find this compression position on yourself. Practice finding this location many times.

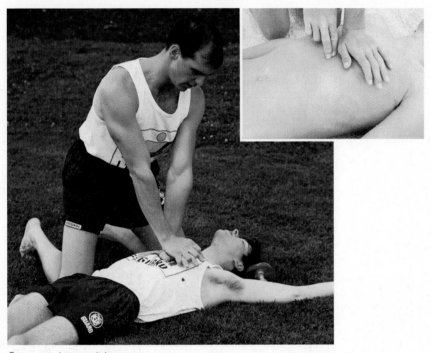

Compression position.

3. Take the heel of the palm of your free hand and place it in the center of the chest directly above (toward the head) your two fingers.

4. Now remove your two fingers and interlock (place) that hand on top of the other hand already in the center of the sternum. If you ever take your hand off the chest wall, you **must** start again and find the correct position.

5. Place your upper body directly over your hands with your shoulders on the same vertical plane as the nose and naval. Lock your arms and only pivot at the hips.

COMPRESSION DEPTH AND RATE

Depth

Chest compressions are performed in an attempt to circulate blood in a closed system by compressing the pump (heart) between the sternum (breastbone) and the bony spinal column. Compressing the heart in this manner only provides the injured guest with 25% of the blood flow normally produced by the healthy beating heart. After confirming proper hand and upper body positions, you must press down on the chest wall approximately 1-1/2 to 2 inches. This depth will usually be between 1/3 and 1/2 of the total chest height. Do not be alarmed if ribs fracture during compressions. Remember, a person who is not breathing and has no pulse is dead, and breaking a few ribs in the attempt to save his or her life is a better thing than death!

Rate

When compressions are in progress, a beneficial compression rate must be maintained. If you compress at a rate too slow, the guest will die. If you compress at a rate too fast, the guest will die, and you will become exhausted quickly. The proper rate allows the heart to adequately refill between compressions. The *Journal of the American Medical Association* (JAMA) recommends a compression rate of 80 to 100 compressions per minute in the adult patient. Simple math reveals that compressions must therefore be performed at a rate faster than 1 per second, so pick up the pace. Counting techniques such as "One Mississippi, Two Mississippi, Three Mississippi" are too slow.

COMPRESSION RATE AND RESCUE BREATHING

A ratio is the comparison of two or more numbers. The ratio of compressions to rescue breaths in adult CPR is 15 compressions for every 2 breaths or 15:2. Every time you complete 15 compressions and 2 breaths a CYCLE is counted. In 1 minute of resuscitation, you should be able to complete 4 cycles.

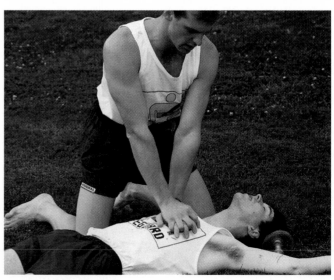

Fifteen compressions.

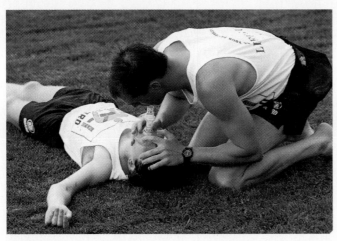

Two breaths.

Every few minutes, or if the guest shows signs of improved consciousness (moaning, moving, etc.) you should immediately check the guest's pulse for 5 to 10 seconds.

If you find a pulse, check the status of the guest's breathing by using the head tilt-chin lift or jaw thrust method and looking, listening, and feeling. If breathing is absent, perform rescue breathing techniques while constantly monitoring the guest's pulse.

If you do not find a pulse, administer two breaths and again begin compressions. Monitor the status of the pulse every few minutes.

Remember to immediately activate the EAS/EMS if the adult patient is unresponsive.

COMMON CPR PERFORMANCE ISSUES

◆ Hand position is incorrect.

◆ Depth of compression is incorrect.

◆ An adequate seal around the nose and mouth is not maintained.

◆ The lifeguard pivots at the elbows or knees during compressions.

◆ Rescue breaths are too forceful.

◆ Proper airway position is not maintained.

◆ The EAS/EMS is not activated soon enough.

◆ Either pulselessness or breathlessness is not recognized.

◆ **Danger:** many patients undergoing CPR will vomit—maintain the airway by rolling the patient on the side and clearing the airway.

TWO-PERSON CPR TECHNIQUES

In many emergency situations, more than one lifeguard first responder will be involved. In CPR events, more than one person can perform the resuscitation skills. The resuscitation hands on skills are similar in two-person resuscitation. The compression to rescue breath ratio changes to 5:1. One person performs chest compressions, while the other person performs the rescue breaths. When either of the first responders becomes tired of their respective skill, a change or shift can be made at the end of the cycle. Begin with a breath and end with a breath prior to any shifting of positions.

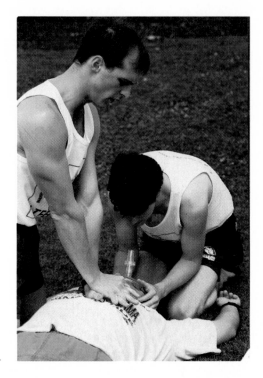

Two-lifeguard CPR.

FOREIGN BODY AIRWAY OBSTRUCTION (FBAO) MANAGEMENT

Occasionally, complete airway obstructions cause unconsciousness and cardiopulmonary arrest. Ironically, the most common cause of upper airway obstruction is unconsciousness and cardiopulmonary arrest. The tongue commonly causes airway obstruction in the unconscious person who has lost muscle control. Upper airway obstruction can also occur from almost any object that can be placed in the mouth. In adults, alcohol consumption is a major factor in airway obstruction. There are two categories of FBAO: partial and complete.

Partial Obstruction

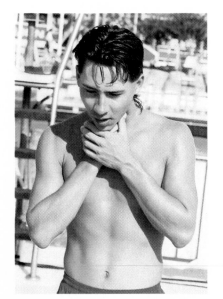

Universal sign of distress: clasping the throat.

A partial airway obstruction will allow the guest some limited air movement and usually stimulate a gag reflex. The guest will be coughing, gagging, and making a forceful attempt at dislodging the object. The guest will appear anxious and frightened and occasionally be clutching the throat.

Treatment of Partial Airway Obstruction

1. Assess the amount of air exchange. Is the gagging and coughing effective? Can the guest make sounds or talk?

2. Reassure the guest and coach her in attempts to dislodge the object naturally.

3. Monitor the guest until the object is removed or the obstruction becomes complete. If the partial obstruction persists, activate the EAS/EMS.

4. Do not attempt to dislodge the object forcefully with back blows or other similar techniques.

Complete Airway Obstruction

A complete airway obstruction is just that—little or no air is able to enter or exit the airway. ***THIS IS A LIFE-THREATENING EMERGENCY!*** The guest will be unable to breath, cough, or talk. The guest's skin color will become cyanotic (blue), especially around the lips and fingers.

Treatment of Complete Airway Obstruction

Conscious Adult

1. If the guest is still conscious, ask "Are you choking?"

2. If the guest is unable to respond, tell him you are going to help dislodge the object using the Heimlich maneuver.

3. Quickly stand behind the guest and wrap your arms around his waist. Support and stabilize yourself to suddenly hold the guest's full weight. Place the thumb side of one fisted hand against the abdomen between the naval and the xiphoid process. Take the other hand and grasp the fisted hand.

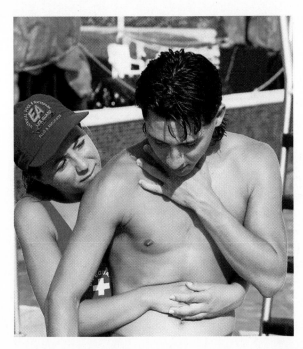

Heimlich position with
conscious adult.

4. Quick, upward thrusts are then performed, pushing the abdomen inward and upward against the diaphragm muscle. The thrusts should be continued until the object is dislodged or the guest becomes unconscious.

5. If the guest becomes unconscious, assist him to the floor, protecting the head and neck from injury. Perform five abdominal thrusts.

6. Open the guest's mouth by grasping the tongue and lower jaw and lifting. Insert the index finger of the other hand along the inside of the cheek deep into the throat. Using a hooking action attempt to remove the object if found.

7. If the guest is having seizures, no attempt at a finger sweep should be made.

Unconscious Adult

1. Activate the EAS/EMS.

2. Perform the primary survey.

3. Attempt to breathe into the guest's airway and reposition the guest if the first attempt fails.

4. If rescue breaths are unsuccessful, straddle the injured guest with your knees aside the guest's thighs. Find the navel and xiphoid process and place your hands between them as shown.

5. Perform up to 5 abdominal thrusts.

6. Finger sweep.

7. Attempt rescue breaths and reposition the guest's airway if necessary.

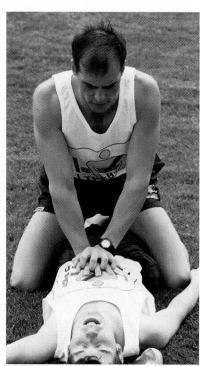

Body and hand position for an unconscious adult with foreign body airway obstruction.

If the airway remains obstructed, continue steps 4 through 7 until the object is dislodged or EAS/EMS arrives.

FBAO in the Pregnant or Obese Person

The FBAO sequences remain the same for pregnant or obese persons; however, the hand position is moved upward to the same location as chest compressions in CPR. Remember that you are trying to create an artificial cough and not squeeze the chest in a "bear hug" style.

CARDIOPULMONARY RESUSCITATION (CHILD)

As the lifeguard first responder you must become familiar with the skills necessary to perform CPR on a child. The American Heart Association offers a guideline which recommends that persons between the ages of 1 year and 8 years be treated as children. This is only a guideline and adjustments must be made for individual children. Have you ever seen an 8-year-old child who was as large as you? Get the point?

Virtually all the CPR and foreign body airway obstruction steps and techniques for the adult are also performed on the child with only minor changes. Here is a comprehensive list of those changes:

Changes to CPR for the Child

◆ If the lifeguard first responder is alone, activation of the EAS/EMS occurs after 1 minute of CPR.

◆ Rescue breath force is reduced appropriate to the child's size (i.e., half a breath).

◆ One rescue breath should take 1 to 1-1/2 seconds to complete.

◆ The mouth-to-barrier mask must be the appropriate size.

◆ Chest compression depth is reduced to 1 to 1-1/2 inches or 1/3 to 1/2 of the total depth of the chest.

◆ Chest compressions should be performed using only the heel of one hand while keeping the other hand on the child's forehead.

◆ Chest compression to rescue breath ratio = 5:1.

◆ Chest compression rate = 100 per minute.

◆ Rescue breathing rate is 1 every 3 seconds or 20 times a minute.

◆ Abdominal thrusts are performed with less force.

◆ Blind finger sweeps are not performed. Visualization of the object is necessary before any attempt to retrieve it with a finger sweep is tried.

CARDIOPULMONARY RESUSCITATION (INFANT)

Cardiopulmonary resuscitation for infants is performed on those between birth and 1 year of age. Lifeguard first responders should remember that this age range is a guideline, and adjustments must be made during the primary survey.

Assessment

The primary survey for infants is altered slightly. If you are alone, EAS/EMS is activated for the unresponsive infant undergoing CPR after 20 cycles or 1 minute. If the infant does not require CPR, then EAS/EMS activation should occur immediately. If possible, and you are alone, transport the infant with you to the nearest telephone.

When assessing the airway (A) of an infant, use the head tilt-chin lift method. Place one hand on the forehead, extending the neck. The index finger of the free hand then lifts the lower jaw by lifting the chin. Care must be taken when opening the infant's airway so as not to hyperextend the neck and "kink" the airway tube. The infant's head is in a "sniffing" position.

Check breathing (B) by looking, listening, and feeling. Pay particular attention to the rise and fall of the abdomen as many infants are "belly breathers." This assessment should take between 3 and 5 seconds. If spontaneous breathing is absent, begin rescue breathing techniques.

RESCUE BREATHING/ARTIFICIAL VENTILATIONS (INFANT)

When performing ventilations on the infant, seal both the mouth and nose with your mouth or the appropriate mouth-to-barrier device. Ventilation volume should be appropriate to the size of the infant (small cheek puffs). The rescue breathing rate for infants is 1 breath every 3 seconds or 20 times every minute. After the airway is open and artificial ventilations are successful, a pulse check is performed by checking the brachial artery.

Assessing the status of the infant's circulation (C) should take between 5 and 10 seconds. If the pulse is absent, begin infant chest compressions in conjunction with artificial ventilations.

CHEST COMPRESSION TECHNIQUES (INFANT)

The area for chest compressions for infants is the lower third of the sternum. In order to find this landmark, draw an imaginary line located between the nipples, directly over the breastbone:

1. Using the index, middle, and ring fingers, place your index finger on the line between the nipples.
2. Center all three fingers directly over the sternum and raise the index finger off the chest.
3. Use the free hand to maintain head position to facilitate breaths.
4. Begin chest compressions at a depth of 1/2 to 1 inch or 1/3 to 1/2 of the total depth of the chest.
5. Use a compression to rescue breath ratio of 5:1 with a rate of at least 100 compressions per minute.
6. If alone, activate EAS/EMS after approximately 1 minute or 20 cycles. If possible, perform CPR while moving the infant to a location where EAS/EMS can be activated.

FOREIGN BODY AIRWAY OBSTRUCTION (INFANT)

Partial Airway Obstruction in a Conscious Infant

Let the infant attempt to dislodge the object naturally.

Complete Airway Obstruction in a Conscious and Unconscious Infant

Many infants will place foreign objects into their mouths. Common objects are coins, peanuts, hard candy, and rocks. When assessing the infant, look for signs or symptoms of anxiety, cyanosis (blue color), ineffective coughing, and altered mental status. Pay particular attention to the infant's surroundings. Are there other objects lying around on the floor that could have been placed into the airway?

Once you have determined that the infant is suffering from a complete airway obstruction, you must act fast:

1. Quickly place the infant in a face down (prone) position over your forearm and place your forearm on the thigh as support. Place your fingers in such a manner as to support the head and not block the airway.

2. Take the heel of the free hand and deliver up to 5 back blows between the infant's shoulder blades. Raise the hand approximately 6 to 10 inches off the back.

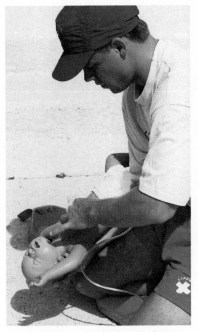

Position for an infant with foreign body airway obstruction.

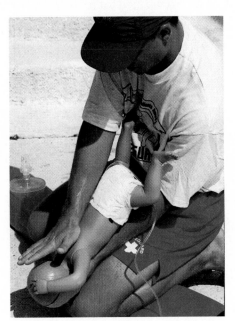

Back blows for an infant.

3. After the back blows, place the free hand on the infant's back and support the head. In this position the infant is effectively sandwiched between your forearms and is ready for re-positioning.

4. Turn the infant into a face-up position (supine) and locate the chest compression landmark. Remember to always keep the infant's head lower than the trunk. Deliver up to five quick chest thrusts in the exact manner as you would deliver chest compressions. If an infant is conscious, keep repeating the back blows and chest thrusts until the object is dislodged or the infant becomes unconscious.

5. If the infant becomes unconscious, place the infant onto a hard surface and open the airway. Activate EMS.

6. Remove any foreign objects that are visualized.

7. Attempt rescue breathing.

8. If the first ventilation is unsuccessful, slightly reposition the head and attempt a second breath. If the airway remains completely obstructed, repeat the sequence of back blows, chest thrusts, and rescue breathing. This process should continue until the object is relieved and ventilations are successful or EAS/EMS arrives.

REVIEW QUESTIONS

1. T F   CPR skills are easy to learn, and if practiced often, easy to recall.

2. Put the following steps in the adult primary survey in order:

   _____   If the guest does not respond, call for help.

   _____   Head-tilt, chin-lift, or jaw thrust.

   _____   Shake and shout, "Are you OK?"

   _____   Look, listen, and feel.

   _____   Check for pulse.

   _____   Give two full breaths.

3. If a guest has a pulse, but is not breathing, you should:

   _____

4. If a guest is breathing on his or her own, you should:

   _____

5. T F   An infant's pulse should be checked at the carotid artery in the neck, for 5–10 seconds.

6. T F   When performing rescue breathing, if a breath does not go in, reposition the head and try again.

7. If repositioning the head does not open an obstructed airway in an adult or child, you should then give _____ abdominal thrusts.

8. Match the rescue breathing rates with the type of guest:

   _____ Infant   a. 1 breath every 5 seconds

   _____ Child   b. 1 breath every 3 seconds

   _____ Adult   c. 1 breath every 3 seconds

9. T F   Counting for the rescue breathing rate should be done out loud and with the count of one one-thousand, two one-thousand, three one-thousand, four one-thousand, **breathe** for an adult.

10. T F   For a person who has an obstructed airway and is conscious, the Heimlich maneuver of grasping around the guest from behind and performing quick, upward abdominal thrusts until the object is dislodged or the guest becomes unconscious is the best method.

SKILL SHEET 7

CPR Review

ITEM	INFANT (0–1 year)	CHILD (1–8 years)	ADULT (>8 years)
How to open airway?	Head-tilt/chin-lift	Head-tilt/chin-lift	Head-tilt/chin-lift
How to check breathing?	Look at chest and listen and feel for air (3–5 seconds)	Look at chest and listen and feel for air (3–5 seconds)	Look at chest and listen and feel for air (3–5 seconds)
What kinds of breaths?	Slow, make chest rise and fall	Slow, make chest rise and fall	Slow, make chest rise and fall
Where to check pulse?	Brachial artery (5–10 seconds)	Carotid artery (5–10 seconds)	Carotid artery (5–10 seconds)
Hand position for chest compressions?	1 finger's width below imaginary line between nipples	1 finger's width above tip of sternum	1 finger's width above tip of sternum
Compress with?	2–3 fingers	Heel of 1 hand	Heels of 2 hands, one hand on top of the other
Compression depth?	1/2–1 inch	1–1-1/2 inches	1-1/2–2 inches
Compression rate?	at least 100+ per minute	100 per minute	80 to 100 per minute
Compression : breath ratio?	5 : 1	5 : 1	15 : 2
How to count for compression rate?	1, 2, 3, 4, 5, breathe	1 and 2 and 3 and 4 and 5 and breathe	1 and 2 and 3 and 4 and and 5 and 6 and . . . 15 and breathe, breathe
How often to reassess?	Every few minutes	Every few minutes	Every few minutes
After reassessment resume CPR with?	Compressions	Compressions	Compressions
How often to give only breaths during rescue breathing?	Every 3 seconds. Count one one-thousand, two one-thousand, (breathe).	Every 3 seconds. Count one one-thousand, two one-thousand, (breathe).	Every 5 seconds. Count one one-thousand, two one-thousand, three one-thousand, four one-thousand (breathe).

SKILL SHEET 7.A: CPR Flow Chart

When actually performing
CPR or Rescue Breathing—
remember to ALWAYS
USE UNIVERSAL
PRECAUTIONS!

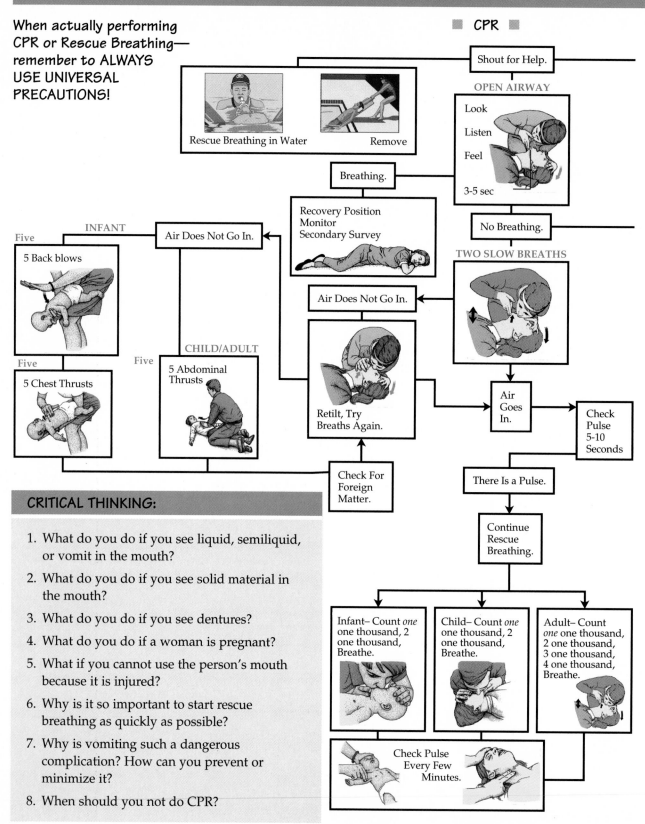

■ CPR ■

Shout for Help.

OPEN AIRWAY

Look
Listen
Feel
3-5 sec

Rescue Breathing in Water   Remove

Breathing.

No Breathing.

Recovery Position
Monitor
Secondary Survey

TWO SLOW BREATHS

INFANT

Five
5 Back blows

Air Does Not Go In.

Air Does Not Go In.

CHILD/ADULT

Five
5 Chest Thrusts

Five
5 Abdominal
Thrusts

Retilt, Try
Breaths Again.

Air
Goes
In.

Check
Pulse
5-10
Seconds

Check For
Foreign
Matter.

There Is a Pulse.

Continue
Rescue
Breathing.

Infant– Count *one*
one thousand, 2
one thousand,
Breathe.

Child– Count *one*
one thousand, 2
one thousand,
Breathe.

Adult– Count
one one thousand,
2 one thousand,
3 one thousand,
4 one thousand,
Breathe.

Check Pulse
Every Few
Minutes.

CRITICAL THINKING:

1. What do you do if you see liquid, semiliquid, or vomit in the mouth?

2. What do you do if you see solid material in the mouth?

3. What do you do if you see dentures?

4. What do you do if a woman is pregnant?

5. What if you cannot use the person's mouth because it is injured?

6. Why is it so important to start rescue breathing as quickly as possible?

7. Why is vomiting such a dangerous complication? How can you prevent or minimize it?

8. When should you not do CPR?

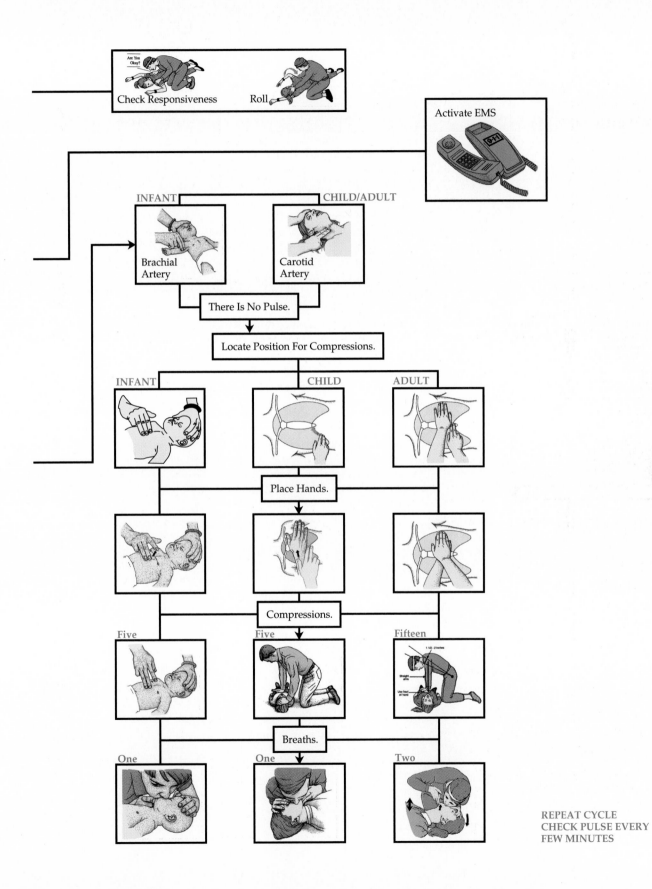

SKILL SHEET 7.B

Two-Rescuer CPR

Entry of Second Trained Rescuer to Perform Two-Rescuer CPR	#1 Performing one-rescuer CPR
	
	#2 Says:
	• "I know CPR"
	• "EMS has been activated"
	• "Can I help?"
	
	#1 • Completes CPR cycle (15 compressions and ends on 2 breaths)
	• Says "take over compressions"
	• Checks pulse and breathing (5 seconds)
	• If pulse absent, #1 rescuer says "no pulse, continue CPR"
	
	#2 • Gives 5 compressions (at 80–100 per minute rate)
	• After every 5th compression, pauses for #1 rescuer to give 1 full breath
	
	#1 • Monitors victim while #2 performs compressions:
	   (a) watches chest rise during breaths
	   (b) feels carotid pulse during compressions
	• Gives 1 full breath after every 5th compression given by #2 rescuer

Two Rescuers Starting CPR at the Same Time	#1 (ventilator) • Assesses victim, if no breaths, gives 2 full breaths; if no pulse, tells #2 to start compressions • Gives 1 full breath after every 5th compression given by #2 #2 (compressor) • Finds hand position and gets ready to give compressions • Gives 5 compressions after #1 says to start them • Pauses after every 5th compression for #1 to give 1 full breath
Switching During Two-Rescuer CPR	#2 (compressor) • Signals when to change by saying "change and, two and, three and, four and, five" or "change on the next breath" • After #1 gives breath, #2 moves to victim's head and completes pulse and breathing check (5 seconds) and if absent says "no pulse, begin CPR." • Gives a full breath after every cycle of 5 compressions #1 (ventilator) • Gives 1 full breath at the end of 5th compression and moves to victim's chest • Finds hand position and gets ready to give compressions • Begins cycles of 5 compressions after every breath
How an Untrained Rescuer Can Help	• Go for help • Monitor pulse and breathing, with some direction • Give CPR with directions (untrained rescuer can learn compressions easier with trained rescuer giving breaths)

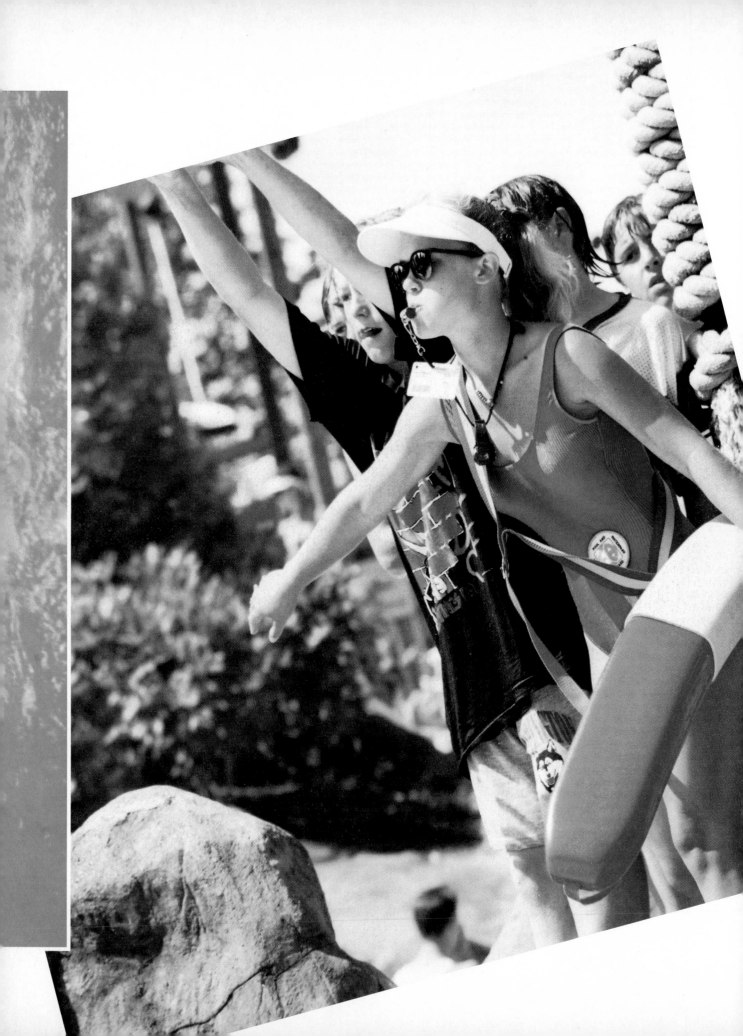

What Do I Need to Do If I Suspect a Spinal Injury?

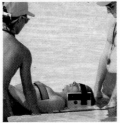

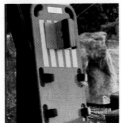

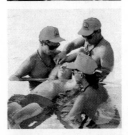

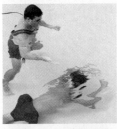

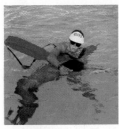

CHAPTER OBJECTIVES

After completing the chapter and related water work, the lifeguard candidate should be able to:

1. Identify situations that might result in spinal injury in the aquatic environment.
2. Identify symptoms of a spinal injury.
3. Perform a no-splash entry and vise grip to minimize risk of further injury.
4. Remove an injured guest from the water using two-lifeguard backboarding.
5. Remove an injured guest from the water using team-lifeguard backboarding.
6. Understand the role of a lifeguard in dealing with a guest with a suspected spinal injury.

When you suspect a spinal injury, you need to use special skills to treat the injured guest. These skills are described in this chapter and should be practiced regularly during your inservice training sessions to maintain your ability to perform these important techniques. You will use these skills any time you **suspect** a spinal injury.

BACKGROUND INFORMATION/SYMPTOMS

Some useful definitions are:

- The **spine** is a column of 33 vertebrae that extend from the base of the head to the tip of the coccyx.

- A **vertebra** is a circular or irregular shaped heavy mass of bone. The side of the vertebra that faces toward the center of the body is the main support of total body weight.

- The **spinal cord** is a cord of nerve tissue contained in the spinal column. All nerves to the trunk, arms, and legs extend from the spinal cord. Unlike many other body parts, the spinal cord cannot be repaired if it is badly damaged. Severe damage to the spinal cord always causes some paralysis.

For every guest suffering a serious head injury, you must assume spinal cord injury. You must not allow the guest to move the neck. The water rescue and subsequent deck treatment must take into consideration the potential spinal injury. Even accidental spinal movement can make the difference between full recovery and total paralysis.

Some signs and symptoms of spinal injury are:

- Pain and tenderness.

- Muscle spasms.

- Paralysis.

- Deformity.

- Bruises and/or cuts on the head or neck.

- Black eyes.

- Altered levels of consciousness (knocked out, garbled speech). **(To date Ellis and Associates clients have never experienced a spinal injury situation where the guest was unconscious.)**

- Vomiting.

- Blood from ears or nose.

When you see these symptoms in a person who has been injured, you should activate the Emergency Action System, call for help, and treat the injured guest according to the training outlined in this chapter. You must become skilled in asking qualifying questions to get enough information from the guest to determine if you should suspect a spinal injury.

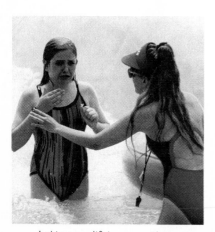

Asking qualifying questions.

SPINAL INJURY IN THE AQUATIC ENVIRONMENT

In the aquatic environment, there are many ways in which a person can injure the spinal column. Some examples include:

- Direct blows to the spine.
- Diving into shallow water.
- Falls from a height.

The only way to find out the extent of a spinal injury is through x-rays. Since you cannot know the extent of injury, you must treat all guests with suspected spinal injuries as if there is spinal cord damage.

As a lifeguard, you can affect the final outcome of the injury. Beginning with the way you enter the water and continuing through all phases of the rescue, you must use extreme care. **You** may make the difference between life and death or life-long paralysis for guests with spinal cord injuries.

SKILLS FOR HANDLING GUESTS WITH SPINAL CORD INJURIES

NPWLTP Position Statement

The National Pool and Waterpark Lifeguard Training Program recognizes the importance of providing care for injured guests suspected of having a spine-related injury while in, on, or about the water. These guests require care that should be provided by medical professionals (EMTs, paramedics, nurses, and/or physicians) who have received extensive training in the proper management of such injuries.

The National Pool and Waterpark Lifeguard Training Program believes that management/treatment devices, such as cervical collars should only be applied by qualified medical professionals who have received extensive training in this specialty. Accordingly, we believe that the role of the lifeguard should be focused on preventing the guest from sustaining further injury until qualified professional medical care is available.

The rescue skills taught in this chapter will minimize the risk of unnecessary movement in the water until a medical professional assumes charge for the care of the patient.

In some instances, it may become necessary to extricate the patient from the water prior to the arrival of a medical professional. The skills taught in this chapter to deal with extrication were designed to minimize the risk of unnecessary movement to guests while removing them from the water when conditions warrant such action. We caution that these skills were not intended to be utilized for the exclusive purpose of spinal injury immobilization and/or treatment. It should always remain the responsibility of the attending medical professional to provide this specialized care.

The care for individuals suspected of having a spinal injury requires well planned protocols. This policy should be developed in joint cooperation with your local EMS provider, aquatic facility administrator, and lifeguard staff. NPWLTP lifeguards should be thoroughly familiar with these protocols and frequently participate in simulated drills to maintain technical competence in the executing of them.

Our safety statistics indicate that the overwhelming number of spinal rescues in the aquatic environment involve conscious and sometimes active guests. While the spinal management skills in this course are generally practiced on simulated unconscious guests to address a catastrophic accident, it is important that you also practice these skills on conscious individuals to gain experience in managing this type of incident. It is important for you to read through the technique descriptions in this chapter both before and after you practice the skills.

While the technical skill execution remains the same under both conditions, additional support is necessary when the guest with the suspected spinal cord injury is conscious. To manage a conscious guest with a suspected spinal injury, additional communication, calmness, and reassurance must be used.

Your spinal injury management begins with the way you enter the water to make the rescue. You must use an entry that does not disturb the surface of the water. When you see an injured guest with a suspected spinal injury, use an ease-in entry: sit on the edge of the pool, and slide in; move toward the guest with no splashing and as little water movement as possible.

The technique you will use while in the water to minimize the risk of unnecessary movement is called the vise grip. You will do this technique using the rescue tube to help hold you and the injured guest on the surface of the water.

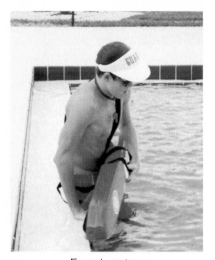

Ease-in entry.

VISE GRIP

The vise grip is an effective method of handling a guest with a suspected neck or spinal injury:

1. Whistle; signal to stop dispatch/waves if necessary; signal for help. Enter the water with an ease-in entry. Slowly approach the injured guest.

2. Position yourself. Stand beside the guest facing in the same direction. Your waist should be in approximately the same area as that of the injured guest. The rescue tube should be between you and the guest, lengthwise along his body. If you are in deep water, you will need to keep your tube across your chest and under your armpits and position yourself higher up next to his body.

3. Use the vise grip. Reach over the guest's body and over the rescue tube with both your hands and place them on the guest's upper arms. Slowly bring the guest's arms up over the head so that the upper arms are pressed firmly about the head near the ear level.

4. **Roll the injured guest.** Roll the guest, **maintaining firm pressure.** Your arms and hands do all the work, while your body stays still. Pull the guest's outside shoulder toward you to begin the roll. Maintain firm pressure on the arms and keep the guest pulled into your body after the roll. The rescue tube will help keep the guest's body floating horizontally and will provide stability for both of you if you are in deep water. Check the guest for breathing and level of consciousness. If the guest is conscious, talk calmly and firmly to her as you make progress toward the backboard or await its arrival. If the guest is not breathing, begin rescue breathing using appropriate techniques. Be sure to keep the guest's face above the water at all times.

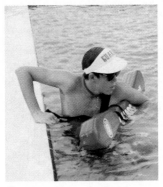 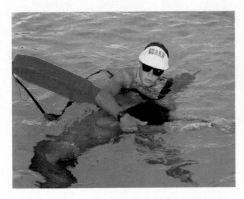 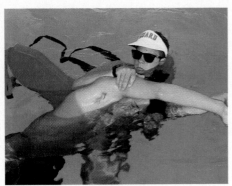

The vise grip.

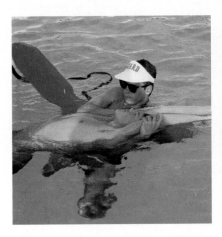 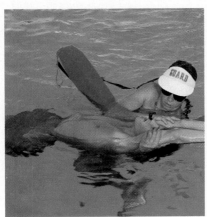 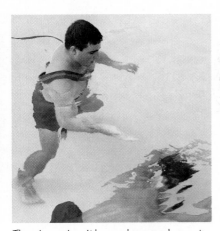

The vise grip with a submerged guest.

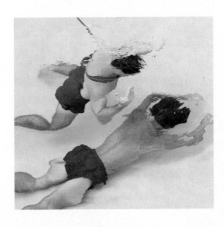 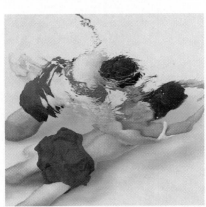 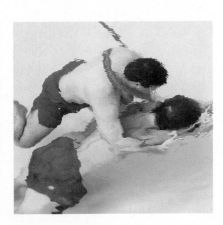

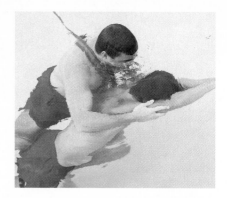
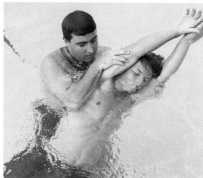
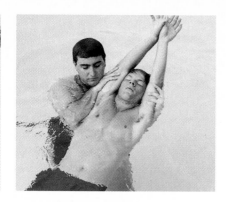

The vise grip can also be used if an injured guest is not in the water, but is on land and showing symptoms of a spinal injury.

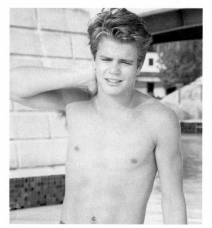

Guests with spine injuries may not always be in the water.

BACKBOARDING

Backboarding is performed by a **lifeguard team,** who will act quickly and efficiently to remove the guest from the water safely. You will learn the procedure for a two-lifeguard team for facilities with a limited number of lifeguards available to assist, and a multi-lifeguard team for facilities that have numerous backup lifeguards available to assist.

It is important that you practice being the initial rescuer, **and** being a member of the support lifeguard team. You need to know what your responsibilities will be in any role on the team.

Backboards, and their accessories, come in many sizes and shapes. You will spend time in training at your facility becoming familiar with your equipment and the team procedure that works best in your situation. Your protocol for spinal injury management will be tailored not only to your equipment, staff size, and facility, but should also involve input from your local emergency medical system providers.

The key components of any backboarding protocol are:

◆ **Communication** between the lifeguard team and with a conscious guest.

◆ **Minimize the risk of unnecessary movement** of the guest throughout the entire backboarding procedure.

◆ **Careful removal** to avoid further injury to the guest or lifeguard.

◆ **Protection from hypothermia** as spinal injury will make a guest more likely to suffer hypothermia, even in warm conditions.

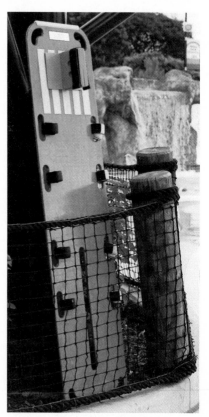

A well-equipped backboard.

TWO-LIFEGUARD TEAM BACKBOARDING

The two-lifeguard team backboarding techniques are performed at the side of the pool. The following steps describe the procedure from the initial recognition of a guest with suspected spinal injury through extrication from the water.

1. Recognize the situation. The first lifeguard whistles, signals the situation, and enters the water, carefully approaching the injured guest. The lifeguard assumes the correct position, performs the vise grip, makes progress toward the pool edge, checks for breathing, and calls out findings. The second lifeguard clears the pool and has 911 called. This lifeguard then brings the backboard to the focal point, removes the blanket and places the head restraints close to the edge, puts the backboard into the water vertically at comfortable arm's reach, and leans on the backboard to keep the end on the bottom. As the first lifeguard approaches with the guest, the second lifeguard slides the backboard under the first lifeguard's foot.

2. Bring the injured guest to the side. The first lifeguard then switches to an overarm vise grip, brings the injured guest to the focal point, and places a foot on the end of the backboard or in the foothold to keep it down.

3. Move the guest to the backboard. The second lifeguard locates the injured guest on the backboard and holds the head by placing the little fingers in the guest's armpit, thumbs out toward sternum, while the inside parts of the wrists and forearms clamp the head. While maintaining even pressure, this lifeguard tells the first lifeguard that the head is secure.

4. Secure the injured guest. The first lifeguard slides her own arms up and out of vise grip (if not already done), lifts her foot off the backboard, and checks the guest's ABC's. This lifeguard then attaches the chest strap, **very tightly high on the guest's chest under the armpits,** regains control of head by placing one hand on the cheekbones, and the other arm under the middle of the backboard, and tells the second lifeguard that the guest is secure.

5. Secure the injured guest's head. The second lifeguard moves hair off the forehead and moves arms down one at a time. This lifeguard then places both head restraints beside the head at the same time, secures the head strap using equal amounts of pressure, continues to hold the restrained head and keep the board stable against the pool edge, and tells the first lifeguard that the guest's head is secure.

6. Use the rescue tube if needed. The first lifeguard may place a rescue tube underneath the backboard for flotation and stability while strapping the guest. This lifeguard secures the next strap loosely across the stomach, firmly secures the next strap across hips or thighs, being careful of the pelvic area, loosely secures legs and feet, reassesses the ABC's, and moves to the feet of the guest.

7. Remove the guest. The first lifeguard in the water lowers the foot end of the backboard while the second lifeguard on deck lifts the head of the board. The water will produce most of the lift so that the second lifeguard does not have to strain to lift the backboard runners onto the edge of the deck. The second lifeguard pulls as the first lifeguard pushes and slides the injured guest and backboard up onto the deck.

8. Care for the guest. Both lifeguards continue to monitor the injured guest. Watch for vomiting. If it occurs, the entire backboard must be

rolled to the side. Do not just turn the guest's head. Remember that a guest without a clear airway, such as one clogged with vomit, will surely die. Cover the injured guest as quickly as possible to prevent hypothermia. Covering can also be initiated in the water with appropriate materials to maintain body warmth if it does not get in the way of the backboarding process.

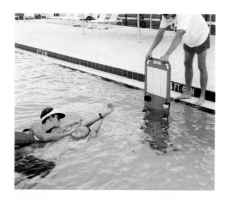 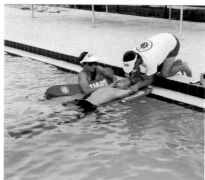 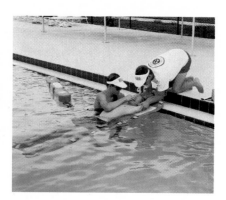

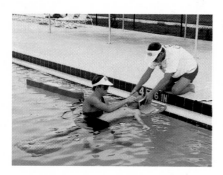 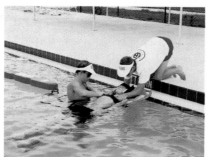 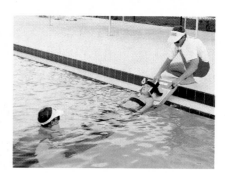

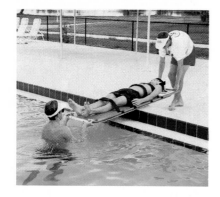

MULTI-LIFEGUARD TEAM BACKBOARDING

The original lifeguard has made the initial rescue and should be talking to the injured guest, assessing ABC's, and communicating to the lifeguard team. By this time, the secondary lifeguard team should have cleared the activity area, have called for emergency personnel, have brought the backboard to the rescue scene, and be ready to assist in placing the injured guest on the backboard. It will also be the responsibility of the secondary lifeguard team to check the guest's ABC's, determine rescue breathing needs, and proceed accordingly:

1. Position the injured guest. While the rescuing lifeguard maintains the vise grip position, other lifeguard team members slowly and gently raise the body of the guest to a horizontal position.

2. Place the backboard. Submerge the backboard so that it is under, but not touching, the guest. Move the backboard so that it is in a centered position underneath the guest.

3. Transfer control of the head. One member of the lifeguard team gets into position near the top of the backboard near the guest's head. This lifeguard holds the head by placing a little finger in the guest's armpit, thumbs toward the sternum, while the inside wrists and fore-arms clamp the head. The pressure should be firm and even. **This lifeguard now assumes control of the rest of the rescue.**

    The original lifeguard's arms and hands are now released out of the vise grip. This lifeguard now becomes a member of the support lifeguard team and assumes a position to the side and continues talking to the guest and/or monitoring the guest's ABC's. After the position change takes place, the backboard is slowly raised underneath the guest.

4. Strap the guest's chest, getting the strap up high above the breast-bone, under the armpits. If the lifeguard is strapping from a vise grip rescue, lower the arms, one at a time, to the guest's side.

5. Place head restraints and head straps.

6. Strap the legs and feet.

7. Remove the guest from the water. Carefully lift the backboard into a level position and carry it to a dry area to await emergency trans-portation.

8. Care for the guest. The original lifeguard continues to monitor the guest's ABC's. Watch for vomiting. If it occurs, the entire backboard must be rolled to the side. Do not just turn the guest's head. Remember that a guest without a clear airway, such as one clogged with vomit, will surely die. Cover the guest as quickly as possible to prevent hypothermia. Covering can also be initiated in the water with appropriate materials to maintain body warmth if it does not get in the way of your boarding process.

    If you are backboarding in deep water, rescue tubes can be inserted under the backboard once it is in position.

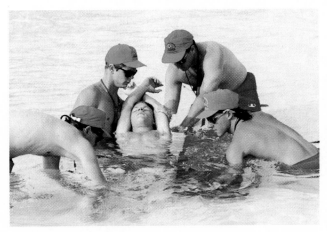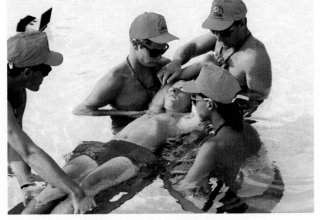

Team lifeguard backboarding.

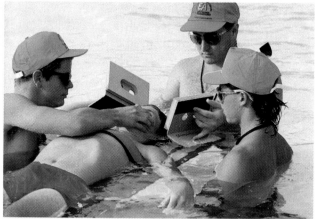

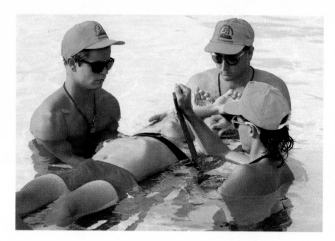

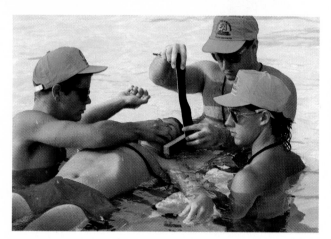

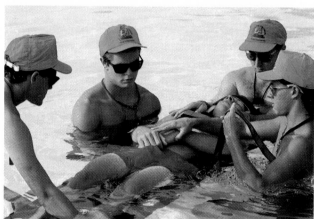

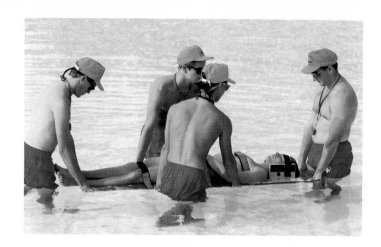

HANDLING SPINAL INJURIES IN SPEED SLIDES

Because of the small space available at the bottom of a speed slide in the run-out, the usual process of managing a suspected spinal injury needs to be modified.

After stopping dispatch and activating the EAS, you will need to apply a vise grip to the injured guest. If the guest is face down, bring them face-up using the vise grip as it would be performed in the water. If the guest is face-up, apply the vise grip hold from the best position to maintain control. This position will depend on the height of the run-out sides, the amount of room inside the slide walls, and other physical features of the area.

When additional lifeguards arrive to help, position them at the side of the slide walls, with equal numbers on each side of the guest. The lifeguards then quickly position their arms over the guest to assure they will be in the correct position, based on the body size of the injured person. The lifeguards should alternate their arms with one another.

The arm/hand positions of the lifeguards should be spaced to provide maximum support along the length of the body, from the shoulders to the feet. Once any position adjustments have been made, the lifeguards place their hands under the guest in the slide run-out, with the lifeguards' arms and elbows inside the walls of the slide.

By this time, the backboard should be in a position inside the slide run-out, at the guests feet. Be sure that all the straps are placed to be clear when the board is positioned under the guest. At your count, and while you maintain the vise grip, the lifeguard team lifts the guest to the top of the slide sides. As the guest is lifted, the other lifeguard team members will slide the board into a position under the guest. You must watch alignment of the board and be sure the guests head will be in a position in the center of the head pad. Communication is very important.

Upon your command, the lifeguard team then lowers the guest to the board. Clear all straps, if they are in the way, and place them on top of the guest. The lifeguard team now gets positioned to lift the board out of the run-out. The lift should be at your command, and lifting should be done with the legs, not the back.

Lift to a complete standing position and stop.

The lifeguard team now rotates the guest and board in a direction that moves the guest's head to the outside of the slide. Movement is done slowly, and allow time for the lifeguard team members to step over the sides of the slide.

Stop when the rotation is complete.

Slowly bring the guest and board down, placing it across the top of the slide sides. Secure the guest to the backboard, monitor breathing, and begin follow-up care according to your emergency action plan.

ADDITIONAL SPINAL INJURY MANAGEMENT ISSUES

If you do not have enough lifeguards available to form your rescue team, and you do not wish to use the two-lifeguard technique, you may use the aid of guests at your facility. You will need to tell them **exactly** what to do. If you use guests to help, **you** are in the role of instructor, teaching them "on the spot" critical procedures.

Recent evidence has revealed that lifeguards execute an alarming number of unnecessary spinal rescues on guests where facts obviously indicated that a different rescue approach should have been used. It is extremely important that spinal management rescues be used only when evidence indicates that such protocols are warranted. For example, an unconscious individual discovered lying on the bottom in 8 feet of water, at the center most point of the pool with no diving board, has no potential to have a spinal accident. Yet, we have discovered that several lifeguards used spinal rescue techniques on individuals who were actually near drowning victims.

Needless to say, better rescue technology is available for unconscious individuals lying on the bottom of the pool than using spinal techniques. You should survey the entire scene of the incident before determining what type of rescue techniques should be used.

REVIEW QUESTIONS

1. T   F   It is not important to talk to a guest with a spinal injury, because he or she will probably be unconscious anyway.

2. T   F   It is your job to prevent further injury to the guest until EMS arrives.

3. T   F   Guests with head or spinal injuries are likely to suffer hypothermia more quickly than usual because of the trauma to their system and should be removed from the water as quickly as possible and kept warm.

4. T   F   The vise grip is a rescue technique used for a guest with a suspected spinal injury . . . with the tube on top of the water, without the tube if a guest is on the bottom.

5. T   F   A compact jump entry is used if a spinal injury is suspected.

6. T   F   You must evaluate each situation carefully to determine if you should suspect a spinal injury, based on the guest's location, activity, and water depth.

SKILL SHEET 8

Vise Grip

1

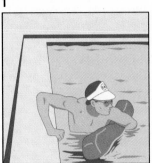

Activate EAS; ease in entry; approach.

2

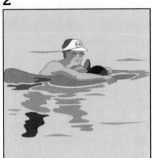

Position; reach over tube and guest.

3

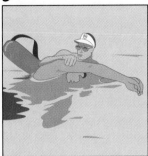

Hands on upper arms; press arms to head.

4

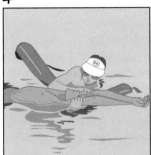

Roll.

5

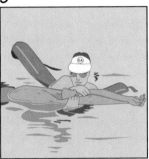

Maintain vise grip; progress to backboard.

6

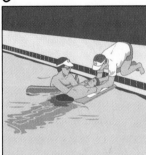

Assess breathing; prepare to use backboard; switch to overarm vise grip.

KEY POINTS:

- Position waist to waist.
- Maintain firm pressure.
- Arms do work, body still on roll.

CRITICAL THINKING:

1. In what situations would this skill be used?
2. How could you do this skill in deep water?
3. What could you do if the injured guest is already face up?
4. How could you perform a vise grip if a guest were a) sitting on the side of the pool, or b) standing?

SKILL SHEET 9

Two-Lifeguard Team Backboarding

1

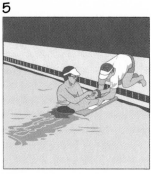

Ease-in entry.

2

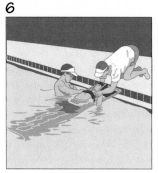

Vise grip.

3

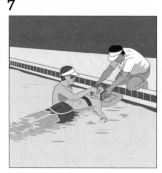

Assess breathing; move guest to side; switch to overarm vise grip (first lifeguard). Slide board in water (second lifeguard).

4

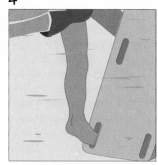

Grab board end with foot (first lifeguard).

5

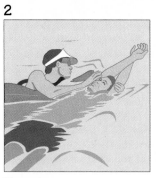

Locate injured guest on board; control head (second lifeguard).

6

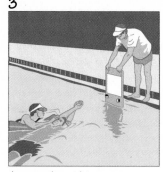

Strap chest; squeeze play around board (first lifeguard).

7

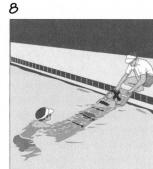

Lower guest's arms; place head restraints; strap head; control head/ stabilize board (second lifeguard).

8

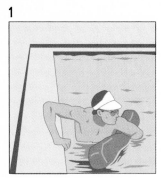

Strap stomach, hips, and feet (first lifeguard).

9

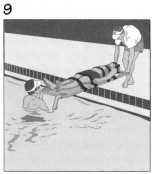

Lower foot end (first lifeguard). Lift head end; slide onto deck; assess/ follow EAS plan (second lifeguard).

SKILL SHEET 9 (continued)

Two-Lifeguard Team Backboarding

KEY POINTS:

- Communicate with conscious guest and with other lifeguards.
- Constantly minimize risk of unnecessary movement.
- Maintain proper board alignment.
- Careful removal of guest.
- Protect guest from hypothermia.

CRITICAL THINKING:

1. If you had to perform this skill in deep water, what could you do to make it work?

Management of a Distressed Guest below the Surface of the Water

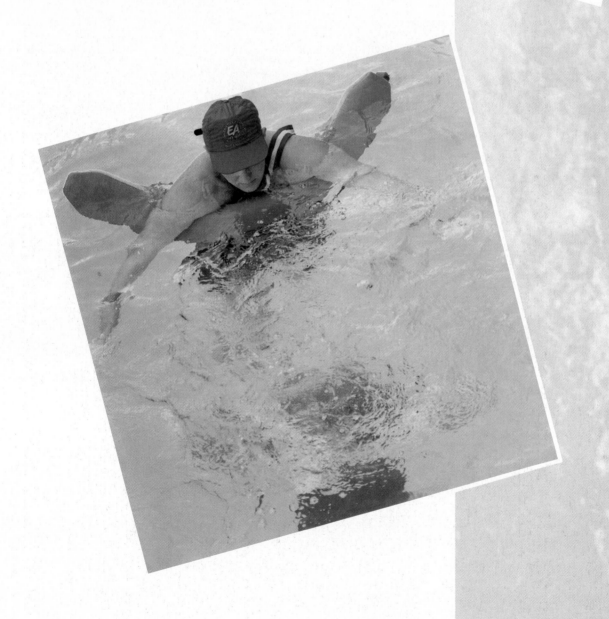

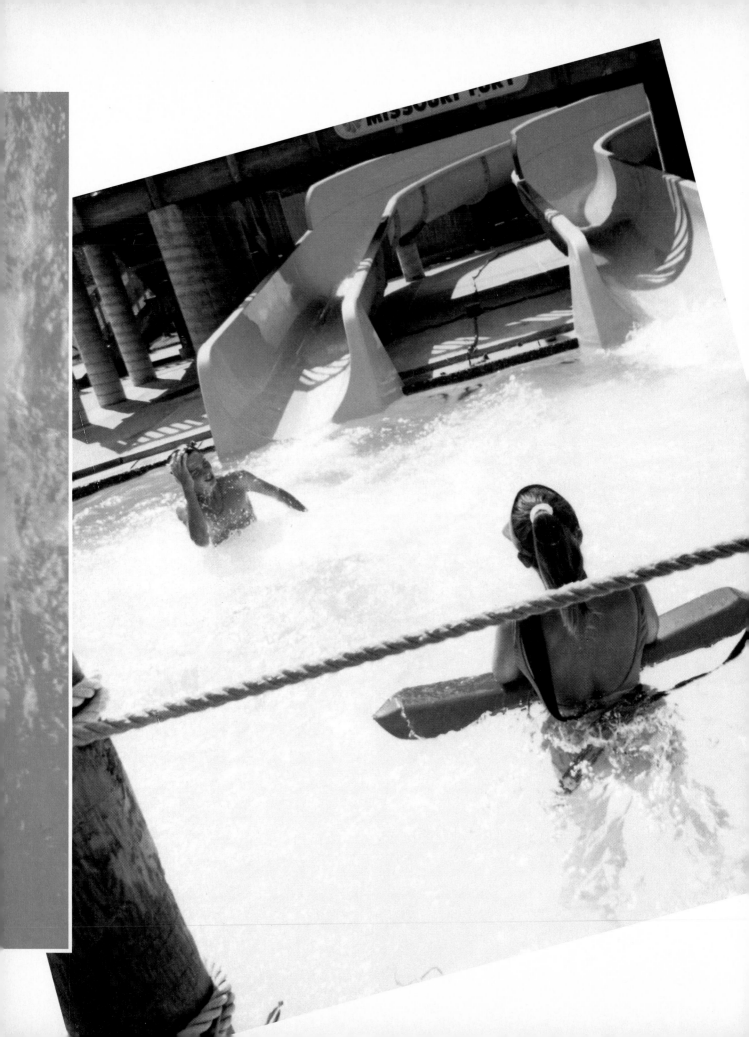

What Do I Do If a Distressed Guest Is within Arm's Reach below the Surface?

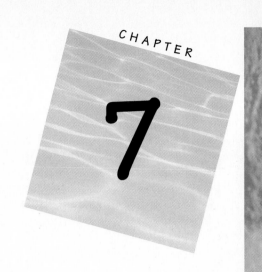

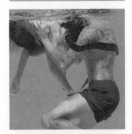
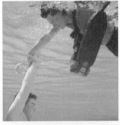
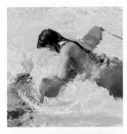
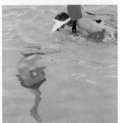
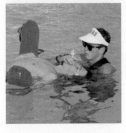

CHAPTER OBJECTIVES

After completing the chapter and related water work, the lifeguard candidate should be able to:

1. Perform a duck pluck on a conscious guest.
2. Perform a duck pluck on an unconscious guest, with follow-up care (CPR).

Many times, a guest in distress will be submerged just a few feet but is unable to get to the surface. The guest may be either conscious or unconscious, and may be either active or passive.

The most effective rescue when a submerged guest is within arm's reach is the "duck pluck." It allows you to remain on the surface of the water, with your rescue tube between you and the guest.

DUCK PLUCK FOR A CONSCIOUS GUEST

1. Whistle, push the E-stop, do a compact jump entry, approach stroke, and stop in front of the distressed guest.

2. Reach across your rescue tube down below the surface and grab the guest's arm. You may need to submerge your head to look down into the water. With your other hand, steady yourself on the rescue tube. It may also be helpful to push your tube down underwater as you make your grab.

3. Pull the distressed guest up, while you drive the tube under the guest's armpit and into his chest. You should be **pushing** the tube with one hand, while you are **pulling** the guest up with the other. This will help keep you from pulling yourself into the guest, or pulling yourself over the top of your rescue tube.

4. Talk to the guest. Keep your arms extended and locked, as you continue to drive forward and make progress toward the side. For added stability of the guest on the tube, you can also wrap the guest's arm over and around the tube and hold it in this position.

5. Secure the guest on the side, assist the guest from the water, and complete the rescue report.

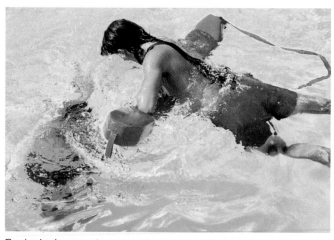

Duck pluck, conscious guest.

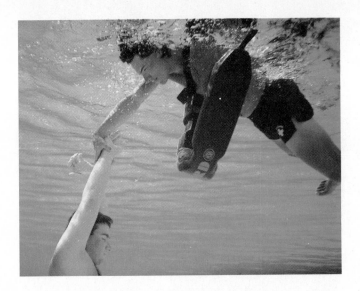

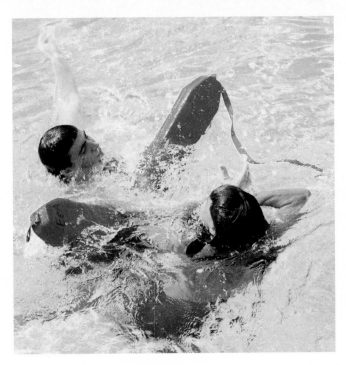

DUCK PLUCK FOR AN UNCONSCIOUS GUEST

1. Execute a duck pluck in the same manner as for a conscious guest.

2. If the guest is unresponsive, grab the shoulder and turn the guest face up so that the rescue tube is underneath the upper back or shoulders.

3. Place guest in the open airway position and begin rescue breathing with a pocket mask.

4. If guest is not breathing, signal for help and begin rescue breathing in the water, using an appropriate pocket mask. Rescue breathing in the

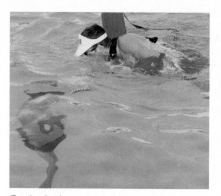
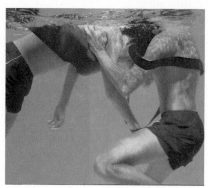

Duck pluck, unconscious guest.

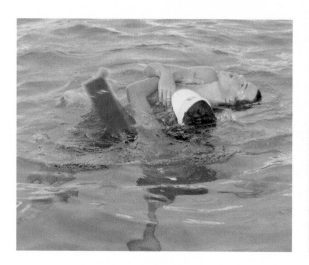
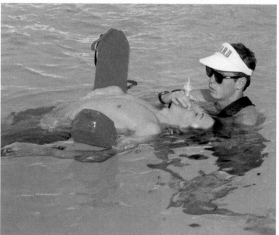

water must be started within the 10/20 Protection Rule, so you must **quickly** get your pocket mask positioned, open the airway, and initiate the first two breaths.

5. Proceed to an exit point and remove the guest from the water, using the best technique for the area in which the incident occurred.

6. Reassess the guest's ABC's, and continue rescue breathing or CPR.

7. Complete the rescue report.

REVIEW QUESTIONS

1. T   F   Many times guests may be submerged just a couple of feet, but they are unable to get to the surface.

2. To help keep you from pulling yourself into the guest or pulling yourself over the top of the rescue tube, you can:

   a.

   b.

   c.

SKILL SHEET 10

Duck Pluck

1
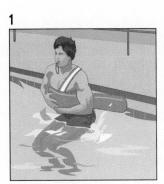
Compact jump.

2
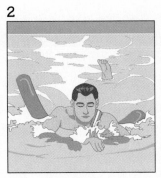
Approach stroke.

3
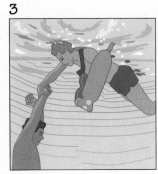
Reach over tube; grab guest's arm.

4
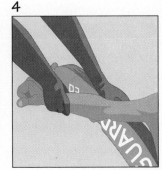
"Push-pull" to get guest up, tube in armpit.

5
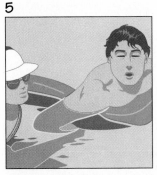
Conscious? Talk; lock arm around tube; kick toward side.

6
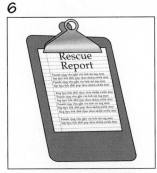
Secure guest; remove guest from pool; complete rescue report.

7
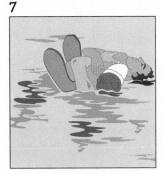
Unconscious? Roll guest, tube under shoulders; open airway.

8
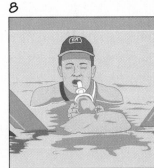
Begin rescue breathing with pocket mask; bring guest to side; extricate guest; assess pulse; follow EAS protocol.

KEY POINTS:

- Keep driving forward.
- Grab and go.
- Keep hips up.
- Submerge tube while grabbing.

CRITICAL THINKING:

1. What if the guest grabs your arm when you reach down to duck pluck?
2. What if you can't reach the guest?

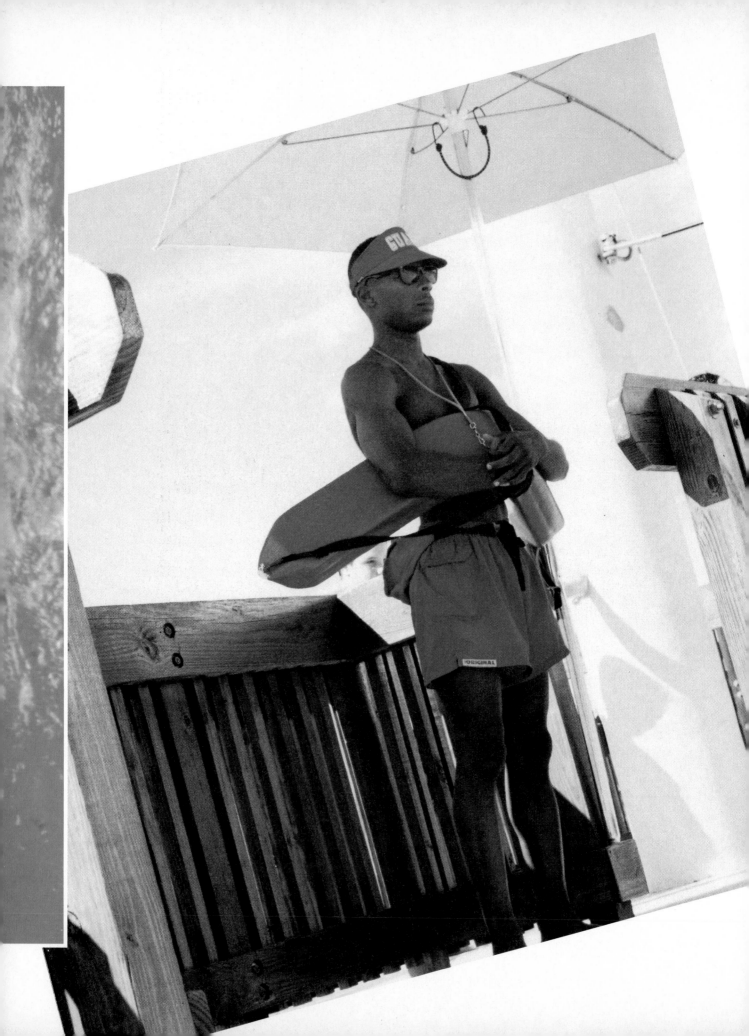

What Do I Need to Do If a Guest Is in Distress below Arm's Reach Underwater?

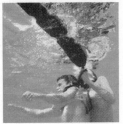

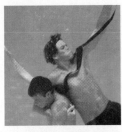

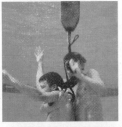

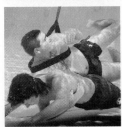

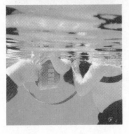

CHAPTER OBJECTIVES

After completing the chapter and related water work, the lifeguard candidate should be able to:

1. Perform a deep water rescue on a conscious guest.
2. Perform a deep water rescue on an unconscious guest, with follow-up care.

A guest who is in distress too far underwater for you to use a duck pluck needs to be managed with special techniques. The guest may be either active or passive, conscious or unconscious, but needs to be returned quickly to the surface.

Your rescue tube will help you bring even a very large guest to the surface. You will use your tube for flotation on the top to help pull you and the distressed guest up to the surface. Once at the top, the rescue tube will be in position for you to manage the rescue.

DEEP WATER RESCUE FOR A CONSCIOUS GUEST

When a guest is unreachable from the surface:

1. Whistle, push the E-stop, do a compact jump entry, approach, stop, and release the rescue tube from under your armpits. Be sure the strap is over your shoulder and across your chest.

2. Do a **feet first** surface dive so that you end up in a position **behind** the guest. While submerging, hold onto the rope of the rescue tube.

3. Roll on your side, in the water, behind the guest. With the arm that is **not** holding onto the rescue tube rope, reach over the guest's shoulder and diagonally across the chest. If possible, get up under the armpit. Your armpit should have strong contact with the guest's shoulder. If the guest struggles, roll with him as you surface. The controlling pressure should be with the arm. While returning to the surface, pull on the rescue tube rope, "feeding" it into your hand that is around the guest. Pull the rescue tube across the guest's chest where he can grab onto it when you break the surface of the water.

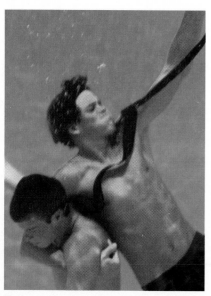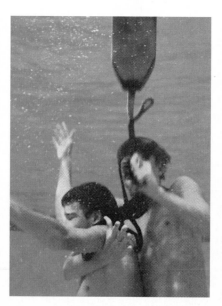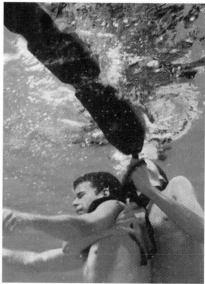

Deep water rescue, conscious guest.

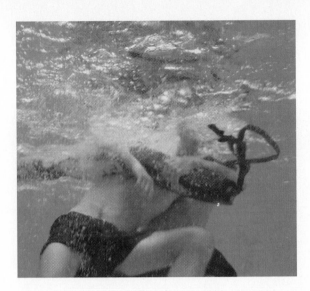

4. When the rescue tube is in place, it should be across the guest's chest with your armpit and the upper portion of your arm securely over the guest's shoulder. The lower portion of your arm should be over the rescue tube pressing it toward the guest's chest, and your hand should be holding the equipment.

   Note: it is important to have the rescue tube across the guest's chest before breaking the surface of the water.
5. Be sure the equipment is secure. Reassure the guest, proceed toward an exit point, secure the guest, provide assistance from the water, and complete the rescue report.

DEEP WATER RESCUE FOR AN UNCONSCIOUS GUEST

If the guest appears to be unconscious when you reach him on the bottom, prepare to put the rescue tube **behind** him rather than in front. This is so you will be in the best position for assessment and rescue breathing when you break the surface.

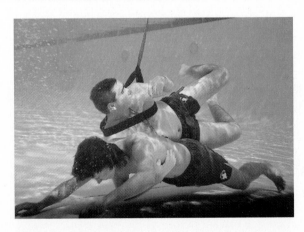

Deep water rescue, unconscious guest.

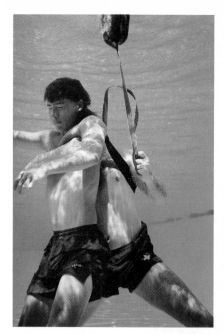

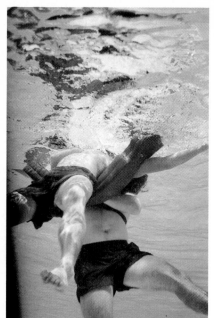

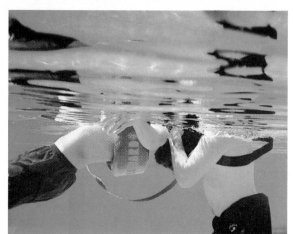

1. When you place the rescue tube **behind** the guest, make sure the guest's airway is in an open position on the tube.

2. If you have your pocket mask, begin rescue breathing. If you do not have a pocket mask, signal for assistance, and await the backup guard who should bring the mask and begin rescue breathing. **Begin rescue breathing as quickly as possible**.

3. Move quickly to a place where you can extricate the guest and give CPR if needed.

REVIEW QUESTIONS

1. T F   In a deep water rescue, your rescue tube will help you bring even a very large guest to the surface.

2. When surface diving to the bottom, you should descend _____ first.

3. After feet first surface diving to the bottom, you should position yourself _____ the guest.

4. If a guest is submerged in deep water and is **conscious,** you will pull the tube _____ of the guest's body when you break the surface of the water. If the guest is **unconscious,** you will pull the tube _____ the guest's body to place the head in an open airway position.

SKILL SHEET 11

Deep Water Rescue

1

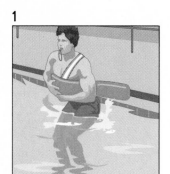

Compact jump entry; approach stroke.

2

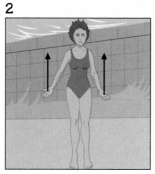

Feet first surface dive to behind guest; hold tube strap.

3

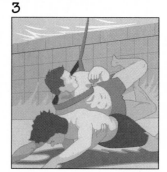

Roll to side; reach across body, hand under armpit.

4

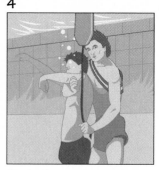

Feed tube strap to other hand while surfacing.

5

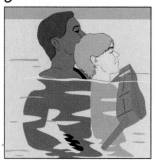

Conscious? Pull tube in front of guest; talk, progress to exit.

6

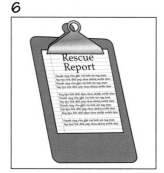

Secure guest; remove guest; complete report.

7

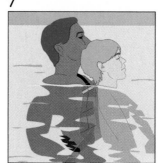

Unconscious? Pull tube behind guest, across shoulders.

8

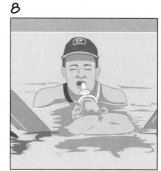

Begin rescue breathing according to protocol; progress to side; extricate guest; assess pulse; perform CPR according to protocol.

KEY POINTS:

- ◆ Have the tube in place before breaking the surface.
- ◆ Pull yourself up to vertical before the feet first surface dive.
- ◆ Use the tube to pull to the surface.

CRITICAL THINKING:

1. What could you do if a guest became unconscious after you had placed the tube in front of him?
2. What could you do if a conscious guest struggles?

Lifeguard Protection

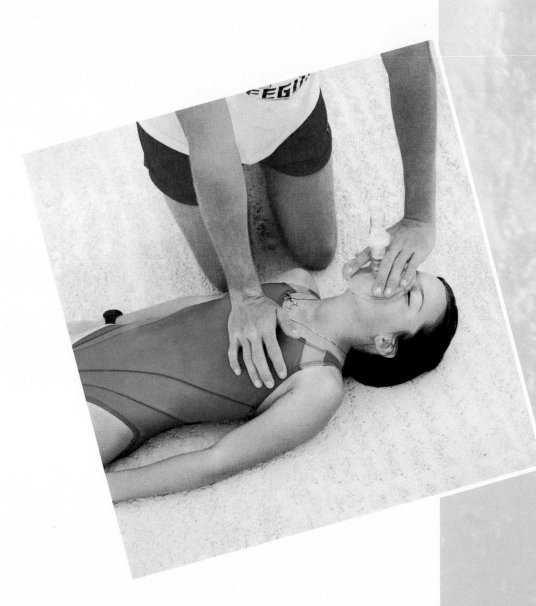

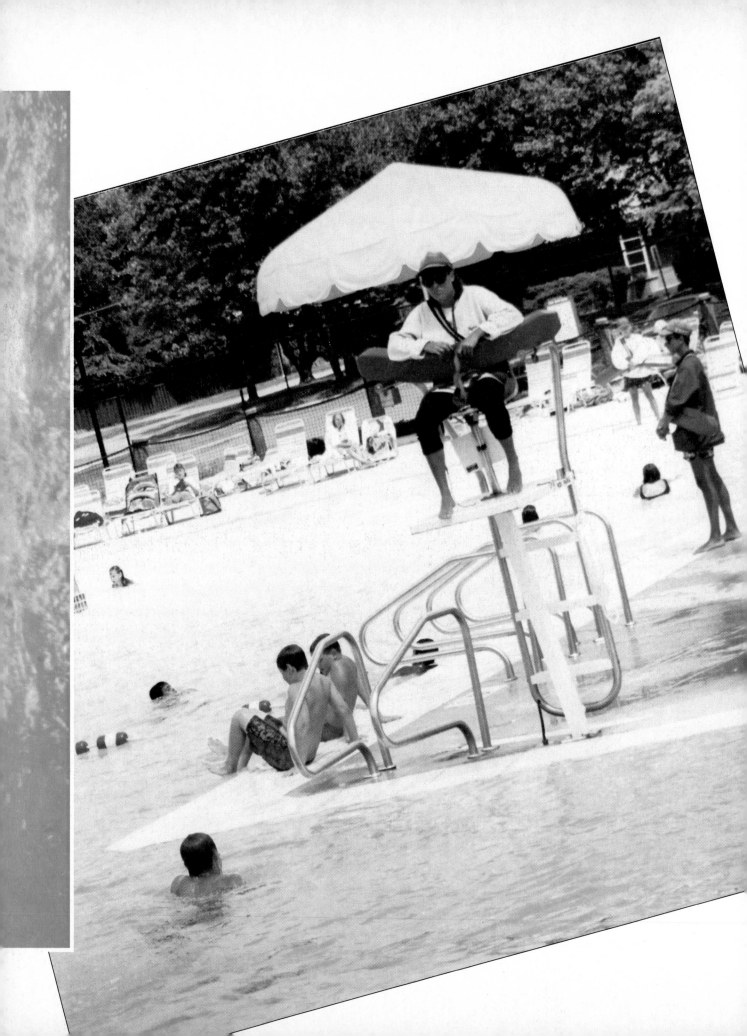

What Do I Need to Do to Protect My Well-Being as a Lifeguard?

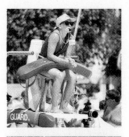

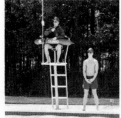

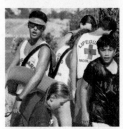

CHAPTER OBJECTIVES

After completing the chapter and related water work, the lifeguard candidate should be able to:

1. List eight health and safety risks you will encounter as a lifeguard and how to reduce those risks.
2. Identify ten strategies for emotionally dealing with being involved in the management of a drowning or a near drowning situation.
3. Understand the concept of legal liability and standard of care.

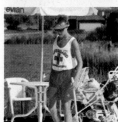

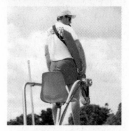

Being a lifeguard can affect your life in many ways. Every day, you are putting yourself at risk, both physically and emotionally. This chapter will discuss some of these risks, and what you can do to protect yourself.

HEALTH RISKS

The health risks you will encounter as a lifeguard, and ways you can protect yourself include:

- Dehydration/heat-related illness—drink plenty of water, use shade, cool down often; **eat sensible, small, light meals.**
- Eye damage—wear polarized ultraviolet protective sunglasses.
- Skin irritation—remove wet suits after work and use talcum powder.
- Skin aging—lubricate skin with moisturizer.
- Exposure to blood-borne pathogens such as human immunodeficiency virus, hepatitis B virus—use Universal Precautions and treat all body fluids as infected.
- Bodily injury or drowning—stay trained: practice your facility's Emergency Action System; practice your rescue techniques; stay in good physical condition; attend in-service training.
- Chemical burns/inhalation—handle any pool chemicals with care, be trained in their use. Be prepared for an emergency.
- Electrical shock—use extreme care when using electrical equipment near the pool. Seek safe shelter when lightning is present.

EMOTIONAL RISKS

In addition to physical risks, you are also putting yourself at risk of experiencing events that could have a tremendous psychological impact

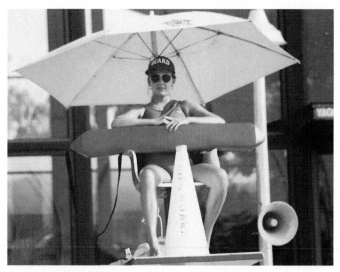

Protect yourself from health risks.

on you. Being the person or a member of the lifeguard team who brings a drowned person to the surface and to the deck is a traumatic experience at the time and can also have some long range effects. Even if you know you did everything correctly and **well,** it is **still** traumatic.

The emotional effects of such an experience can never be completely eliminated, but there are things you can do that will reduce them:

◆ Fill out your report accurately and completely; it's part of doing your job well.

◆ As soon as possible, get in the water and have a workout.

◆ Think about what happened and emphasize in your own mind those things you did correctly and well.

◆ Even though you did everything as well as possible, the questioning session with authorities could be frightening. Just remember that it's a necessary part of "the system."

◆ Remember, guilt is the least beneficial of all human emotions. Put the incident behind you.

◆ Be prepared for media coverage that will probably distort at least some of the facts. Don't let it bother you . . . you know what really happened. Putting yourself on the defensive can be very frustrating and emotionally draining.

◆ Hang in there! Keep up your school work; keep up your job. Those familiar things help, and they are important to you.

◆ Remember, it is important for you to be supportive of the other members of your lifeguard team. They are going through the same type of experience. Don't be afraid to ask for their support, either.

◆ Take advantage of trained individuals in your area who can help you and your lifeguard team deal with stress after you have been involved in a catastrophic incident.

◆ Realize that you won't ever forget what happened. But that doesn't mean that you have to keep remembering it.

LEGAL RISKS

If you are a lifeguard, there is always the possibility of being involved in a drowning incident. If there is a law suit over the incident, it will not be something that is quickly resolved, and your own involvement could be time consuming. (Most litigation lasts 2 to 5 years in this country.) Involvement in litigation could have a serious impact on your future, especially if you are in college or the military or just entering a career field. Litigation can also result in financial disaster.

Is safety maintained because of fear of a lawsuit? While many people believe that society has gone "lawsuit crazy" over the past few years, society would be in much greater difficulty if we did not have a judicial system. The system does need changes and improvements.

However, remember that the system was designed to protect the welfare of each and every citizen.

Society has a right to expect that people will be adequately protected by competent and attentive lifeguards while they are swimming at public facilities. It is disturbing that some people in the industry suggest that the only reason safety is a priority is to protect themselves from a lawsuit. If you recognize this attitude as existing in society today, then you can understand why it is important to believe in and fully support civil jurisprudence. The future of the aquatic industry (and many other things) would be in jeopardy if such a system were not in place. It is true that providing a "reasonable standard of care" is costly. However, the cost of **not** providing a reasonable standard of care is beyond measure, when weighed against the lives and welfare of people in general.

As a lifeguard, you assume responsibility for guest safety and for maintaining a reasonable standard of care. If you are required to render aid, it must be done promptly and efficiently without endangering the guest, other swimmers, or you.

Performance during your rescue attempts will be measured according to *reasonable standards of care* currently expected of the aquatic industry. These standards would be the skills and care that would normally be known and done by others working as professional lifeguards in the same position.

Be aware, however, that your actions when giving follow-up aid such as basic life support and CPR will be measured against that of *health care professionals*. This is because lifeguards are categorized by Department of Labor, the American Red Cross, and the American Heart Association as "health care professionals," meaning that as a lifeguard you will be held accountable for performing technical skills as would paramedics, emergency medical technicians, and other professionals.

The word "professional" in both cases is significant. Society has two different views of lifeguards. The first view is that of a young person who is physically fit, enjoys getting a suntan, and is active among peers: a "fun in the sun" person taking a seasonal or part-time job to help get through school. The second view is usually taken after a catastrophic accident involving a lifeguard. In this view, society takes on the role of judge and jury, asking questions like "How could such an accident occur?", "What were the lifeguards doing?", "Why were the lifeguards unable to perform their lifesaving duties correctly?", etc. In effect, they are asking, did the lifeguard act **professionally** during the emergency? Society expects the lifeguard to be a professional in the way duties are performed and the way an emergency is handled, regardless of what their views are about lifeguards.

The best way to protect yourself from legal liability is to be attentive, conscientious, efficient, and skilled.

Many lifeguards who have been involved in liability litigation were unable to establish their attentiveness prior to the accident and often were unable to confirm basic facts. For instance, many lifeguards could not remember the date and location of their lifeguarding course or the name of their lifeguarding instructor. This makes one wonder just how well they remembered what to do when responding to an emer gency. By actively maintaining the 10/20 Protection Rule at all times when you are lifeguarding, you can establish the level of your attentiveness.

Many lifeguards are also unable to establish their skill level at the time of an incident. The last documented time these lifeguards performed a skill may have been in their training course months prior to an incident. The records of in-service training will show that you are maintaining your skills. Competency is directly related to reinforcement of skills through practice. **At least 4 hours per month should be spent in in-service training.** This time can be scheduled according to what works best at your facility.

In summary, as a lifeguard concerned with liability risk, you:

- Must assume responsibility for guest safety.
- Are held accountable to reasonable standards of care as a health care professional.
- Must be properly trained and maintain your skills through documented regular in-service training.
- Should consider the consequences of litigation and its impact on your future.
- Must act maturely even while associating with and confronting people your own age.
- Must accept potential risk to your personal safety.

REVIEW QUESTIONS

1. For each of the physical conditions listed, name one action you can take to minimize the effects.
   a. Dehydration _____
   b. Skin damage _____
   c. Eye damage _____
2. T F Standard of Care refers to the skills and care that would normally be known and done by others working as professional lifeguards in the same position.
3. T F If you are involved in a lawsuit, it could take many years and be financially draining.
4. T F In-service training should be held 1 hour per month.
5. T T The best way to protect yourself from legal liability is to be attentive, conscientious, efficient, and skilled.
6. List a minimum of four things you can do to reduce the emotional effects of being involved in a near-drowning rescue.
   a.
   b.
   c.
   d.

SKILL SHEET 12

Sun Protection

1

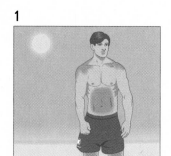

The sun's damage is worse for people with light complexions (red hair, blue eyes, fair skin, etc.)

2

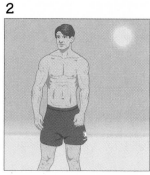

Skin ages prematurely when you don't take good care of it!

3

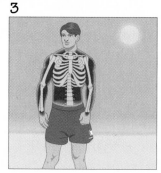

The sun's rays can affect your skin like an X-ray!

4

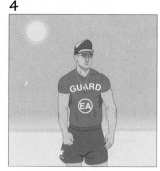

A professional guard wears a hat, shirt, glasses and SPF-15 sunscreen!

5

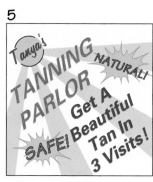

There is no such thing as a safe tanning parlor!

As a lifeguard, **you have to take care of your skin** from the possible dangerous effects of too much sun.

The sun is a source of radiation (UV-A or UV-B rays). The radiation is similar to that of X-rays in that the harmful effects are cumulative and can manifest 10–30 years later in the form of skin cancer.

The professional lifeguard self-protects him- or herself by using SPF-15 or higher sunscreen whenever in the sun. Additionally, hats or umbrellas and sunglasses are mandatory to protect the nose, forehead, lips and eyes. The best hats have wraparound brims that protect the ears and neck.

Premature aging of the skin (that leathery, wrinkled skin you see on older people from too much sun exposure) is an undesirable characteristic that affects your looks and self-esteem in later years. **Avoid prematurely aged skin and skin cancer. Cover up and use SPF-15 or higher sunscreen when outdoors!**

Lifeguard First Responder

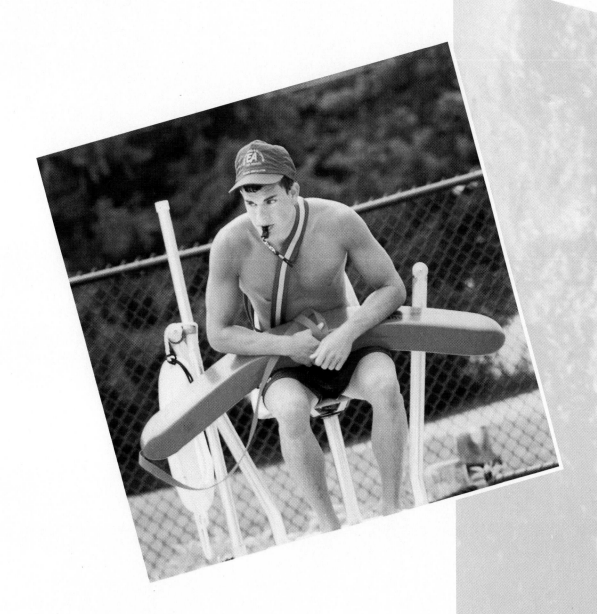

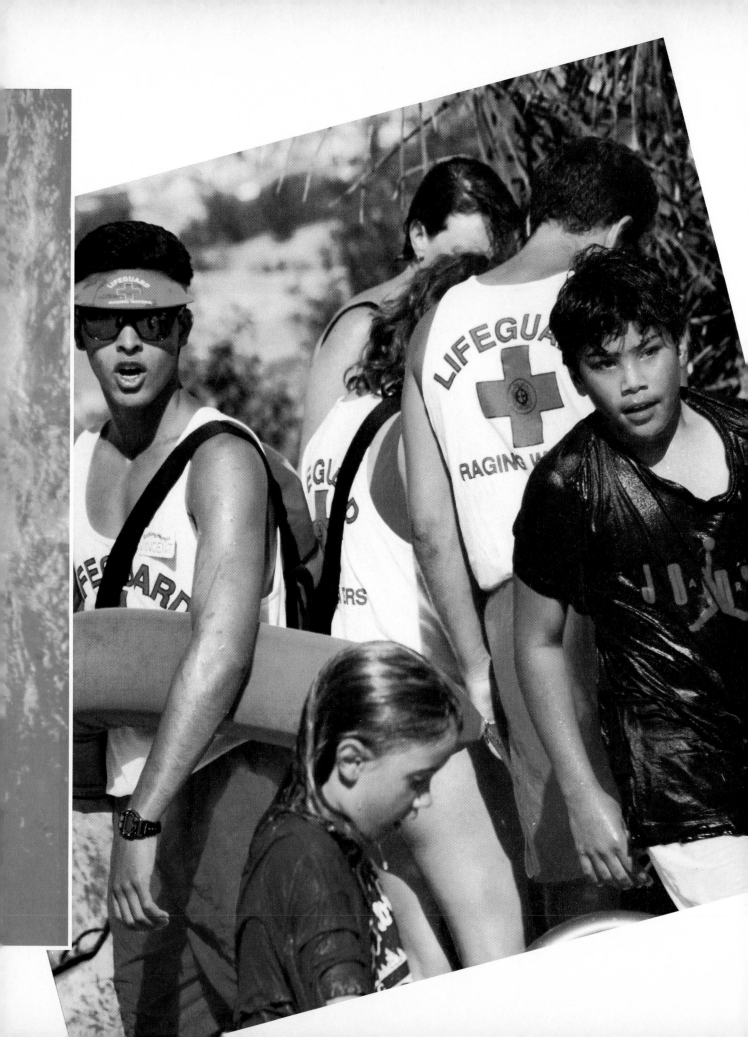

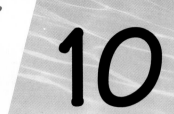

10

What Do I Do If a Guest Has a Nonaquatic Emergency at My Facility?

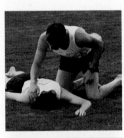

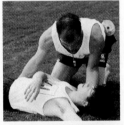

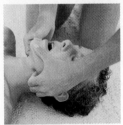

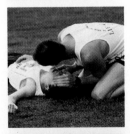

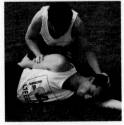

CHAPTER OBJECTIVES

After completing the chapter and related water work, the lifeguard candidate should be able to:

1. Understand your role as a lifeguard first responder.
2. Perform patient assessment—primary and secondary surveys.
3. Identify the symptoms of seven major types of life-threatening emergencies lifeguards are most likely to come in contact with.
4. Identify procedures for managing those seven types of emergencies until EMS arrives.

Unfortunately some professional lifeguards mistakenly believe that as first responders they are sufficiently trained to adequately replace the Emergency Action System (EAS) and the Emergency Medical Services System (EMS). This attitude is incorrect and occasionally leads to additional injury to the already injured guest. Each lifeguard must possess the ability to quickly determine when the EAS/EMS should be activated and the basic "hands on" skills necessary to maintain life until more advanced personnel with training arrive and begin patient care.

This chapter presents only very basic first aid knowledge. Additional first aid information not absolutely necessary during those first few minutes of a medical emergency has been deleted for clarity. Our objective here is to reinforce only the medical information and skills necessary for the lifeguard first responder during first few minutes. This information is not intended to replace more advanced training potentially offered by your aquatic facility. Despite the basic nature of this material, each lifeguard first responder should understand that basic skills if not performed could lead to additional injury and possible death for the guest. Every lifeguard first responder must believe that his or her emergency actions will make a positive difference for the injured guest. You must take your first responder role very seriously.

THE LIFEGUARD FIRST RESPONDER'S RESPONSIBILITIES

The lifeguard first responder's primary responsibilities are:

◆ Recognize aquatic emergencies.

◆ Recognize when to activate the EAS/EMS.

◆ Rescue the injured guest safely and appropriately.

◆ Provide appropriate basic life support and emergency first aid.

◆ Work as a team player in every emergency situation.

◆ Provide the EMS professionals with critical information regarding the emergency event.

Each facility will have specific policies and procedures for activating the EAS, accessing the local EMS system, and handling facility emergencies. As the lifeguard first responder you must become very familiar with these procedures. Learning this information for the first time during an actual emergency can place you and your employer in grave legal danger. Remember, highly trained professionals are just a quick phone call away. In almost every emergency situation, the lifeguard first responder should activate the EAS/EMS and then render competent basic care to the injured guest. Let the EMS professionals do the more advanced care upon their arrival.

Additional lifeguard first responder responsibilities might include:

◆ Train new staff members in EAS/EMS policies and procedures.

◆ Maintain a safe working environment.

- Document rescue/emergency events.
- Continue training and practice in first aid skills.
- Develop injury prevention programs for guest and employees.
- Purchase and maintain basic rescue and first aid equipment.
- Investigate rescue events.

LIFE-THREATENING EMERGENCIES

To define or list all those potential emergencies that qualify as "life-threatening" would take several pages and most likely confuse more than clarify the issue for the first responder.

The lifeguard first responder will define emergencies as life-threatening if the injured guest's airway, breathing, or circulation (pulse) is compromised in any manner. This definition also includes those situations where hemorrhaging (massive bleeding) is found.

INJURED GUEST ASSESSMENT

Objectives of injured guest assessment are:

- Identify and perform the components of the primary survey.
- Understand the importance of maintaining the airway, breathing, and circulation of an unresponsive injured guest.
- Perform a complete secondary survey.
- Identify the proper sequence for activating the EAS/EMS.

Regardless of the first aid emergency, every potential injured guest must receive a complete injured guest assessment. The assessment is divided into two parts: the primary survey and the secondary survey. The primary survey immediately checks for conditions that are life-threatening. The secondary survey commonly reveals conditions or problems which, while potentially serious, can wait minutes or hours for treatment. The injured guest assessment skills are the foundation for all other first aid/CPR techniques. Without a rapid and careful primary assessment, followed by a thorough secondary survey, the lifeguard first responder could be treating the most obvious problem(s) and unfortunately neglecting the less obvious life-threatening conditions. Remember that no matter what the emergency situation, all injured guests must first receive a primary survey.

Components of the Primary Survey (Assessment)

1. Determine the safety of the scene. (Is the area safe to enter; could I be injured by entering?)
2. Determine the injured guest's level of consciousness. (Shake and shout, "Are you OK?")

3. Activate the EAS/EMS immediately if the injured guest is unresponsive.

4. Check the A, B, C, and H of the primary survey:
A = Airway, B = Breathing, C = Circulation, H = Hemorrhaging.

As a lifeguard first responder, you must always be concerned with your own safety first. Never attempt a rescue that will injure you or complicate the emergency situation. If the emergency involves electricity, gases, violence, or other hazardous elements, wait until the proper authorities arrive and secure the emergency scene. Remember a dead or injured lifeguard first responder just complicates the emergency.

When you are able to access (rescue) the injured guest, you must quickly determine the injured guest's level of consciousness. This is accomplished by gently shaking and shouting. If the injured guest does not respond, you must immediately activate the EAS/EMS.

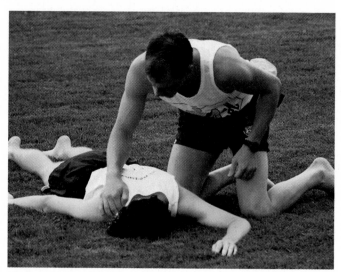

Shake and shout.

An open and clear airway (A) allows oxygen to be delivered to the brain. Any disruption in the airway passage can worsen the injured guest's condition and rapidly lead to irreversible brain damage and death. Keeping this in mind, the lifeguard first responder can understand why the airway becomes so important in **all** emergency first aid/CPR situations. In certain emergency situations you may only be able to maintain a clear airway until the Emergency Action System/EMS team arrives. While this may not seem like much, by maintaining an open airway you have directly influenced the injured guest's chances of survival.

The injured guest's airway (A) can be opened using one of two techniques:

1. The head tilt-chin lift is accomplished by placing one hand on the injured guest's forehead and two fingers on the bony part of the chin. Tilt or bend the forehead back while simultaneously lifting the chin.

2. The jaw thrust is used in injured guests with suspected neck or spinal injuries. The jaw thrust is accomplished by grasping the jaw bone below each ear and lifting up.

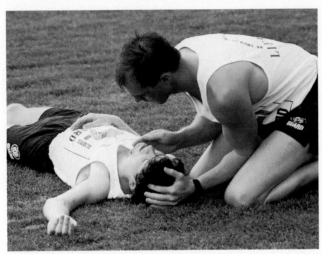
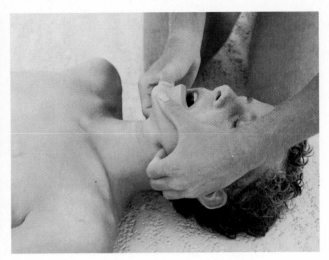

Head-tilt/chin-lift.

Jaw thrust.

Breathing (B) is assessed by placing your head and face down very close to the injured guest's mouth and nose. You must look at the chest and listen and feel for breathing. This should take no longer than 3 to 5 seconds. If the injured guest has stopped breathing, you must begin rescue breathing procedures. As highly skilled lifeguards, you will usually begin rescue breathing/ventilations while still removing the injured guest from the water; an airway mask appropriate for water rescue breathing/CPR situations should be used. You must become very

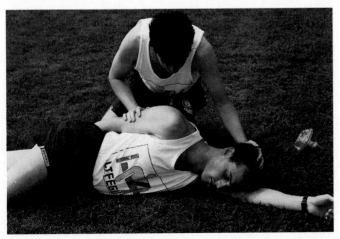

Breathing assessment.

familiar with the application and use of these airway devices. Practice is the only acceptable method to maintain a high level of skill proficiency.

     After assessing the injured guest for breathing (B), check the status of the circulation (C) or pulse. This circulation assessment should take between 5 and 10 seconds. If the injured guest has lost a pulse you must begin the appropriate CPR sequence.

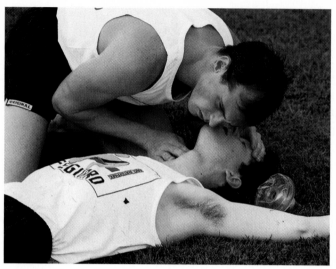

Pulse check.

Injured guests can be breathless and still have a pulse.
Injured guests without a pulse will also be breathless.

     Occasionally you will encounter injured guests who are actively bleeding or hemorrhaging (H). If significant bleeding is found during your primary survey, you must immediately apply direct pressure over the wound area. If possible, the area should be simultaneously elevated above the level of the heart.

Secondary Survey (Head to Toe Assessment)

Only after the primary survey is completed and all life-threatening problems have been treated, should the lifeguard first responder perform a secondary survey. Remember, at no time should you perform a secondary survey while problems still exist with the primary survey's A, B, C, and H. The secondary survey requires the lifeguard first responder to quickly look for and feel for additional injuries. Starting at the head and ending at the toes, look and feel for areas of pain/tenderness, obvious injury/deformity, bruising, etc. During this assessment, constantly communicate with the injured guest, asking about the chief complaint (biggest problem), medical history (i.e., heart conditions, diabetes), and other necessary information. Be sure to relate all this valuable information to the EAS/EMS team leaders.

HEAD, EYE, AND DENTAL INJURIES

Objectives

◆ Recognize the signs and symptoms of serious head injuries.

◆ Recognize the signs and symptoms of serious eye injuries.

◆ Demonstrate the skills necessary to manage a guest with a head or eye injury.

◆ Demonstrate the skills necessary to manage a guest with a dental injury.

HEAD INJURIES

Chapter 6 dealt with head and suspected spinal injury that occurs in the water. You learned about your role as a lifeguard first responder to minimize the movement of the body and head. You also learned special techniques for removing a guest with a suspected spinal injury from the water.

Head and suspected spinal injuries can also occur at your facility outside of the water. The symptoms remain the same, and your role as a lifeguard first responder remains the same with the exception of not having to remove the guest from the water. With every guest suffering a head injury, you should assume accompanying spinal cord injury.

Your primary goal is to maintain the A, B, C, & H, while simultaneously minimizing the movement of the body and head. A vise grip on land should be performed and maintained until EMS arrives.

When dealing with any injury to the head, neck, face or jaw area that has been strong enough to cause distress, be sure to determine how the injury occurred and how much force was involved. Facial and throat injuries can lead to airway obstruction and spinal injury.

EYE INJURIES

Eyes can become injured by a blow, an imbedded object, exposure to chemicals or other substances that can scratch or irritate them. Blindness can result from serious eye injuries.

Signs and Symptoms

◆ Pain.

◆ Redness.

◆ Burning.

- ◆ Headache.
- ◆ Tears.
- ◆ An obvious object in the eye.
- ◆ Loss of vision.

Emergency Treatment for Eye Injuries:

1. If a chemical is in the eye, immediately flush with clean warm water for 15 minutes. Loosely cover both eyes, and seek medical attention.

2. If an object is imbedded in the eye, do not attempt to remove it. Activate the EMS system. Place a protective cup over the eye, and loosely cover the uninjured eye with a dressing and tape both into place.

3. If the eye has received a blow or blunt injury and is not cut, lie the guest on their back with eyes closed. Gently apply a cold pack, and seek medical attention.

4. If the eye area has received a cut, avoid applying pressure. Keep the guest in a semi-sitting position and cover both eyes with gauze pads. Seek medical attention.

DENTAL INJURIES

The dental injuries that may require the attention of a lifeguard first responder will usually involve a broken tooth or a tooth that has been knocked out:

Emergency Treatment for Dental Injuries:

1. If a tooth is broken or chipped, rinse the mouth with warm water. Use a cold pack on the outside of the cheek, and seek attention from a dentist.

2. If the tooth is knocked out, locate the tooth and put it in milk. Seek attention from a dentist as quickly as possible, taking the milk and tooth along.

BURN EMERGENCIES

Objectives

- ◆ Identify the characteristics of first, second, and third degree burns and understand the proper treatment for each.
- ◆ Recognize the signs and symptoms of inhalation injuries and perform the proper emergency treatment.
- ◆ Understand and perform the proper emergency care for dry and liquid chemical burns to the body and eyes.

◆ Perform the proper emergency treatment for the injured guest with electrical burns.

Causes

The burns are divided into three distinct categories: **thermal** burns are caused by contact with flames, super-heated air (steam), radiation (sun), and scalding water; **chemical** burns occur after exposure to dry, liquid, or chemical gases; **electrical** burns are caused by electrocution and lightning.

Degrees of Severity

Burns are also classified according to the degree of tissue destruction. There are currently three distinct degrees: first, second, and third. The lifeguard first responder should remember that many burns include all three levels of severity in same burn area. If you encounter this situation, treat the area according to the highest severity level.

First Degree Burns.   First degree burns affect only the outer layers of the skin, usually turning the skin red and causing slight swelling. First degree burns are very painful and if large portions of the body are affected, the injured guest should seek immediate medical attention. As the lifeguard first responder, you will see numerous guests with first degree burns. Most of these burns will be minor; however, others could be potentially dangerous.

Emergency Treatment for First Degree Burns:

1. If the burn does not cover more than 20% of the body surface area, place the affected area in cool water until the pain stops.
2. If the pain continues suggest that the injured guest contact his or her private physician.

Second Degree Burns.   Second degree burns continue to damage deeper layers of the skin and by so doing cause blisters to appear on the skin. These blisters range in size. In some instances, one blister can cover a large area. The pain will be extreme, and movement usually causes the blisters to break.

Emergency Treatment for Second Degree Burns:

1. After determining and controlling the injured guest's primary A, B, C, and H stop the burning process.
2. If the burn does not cover more than 20–30% of the body surface area, cover the burn area with moist, clean sheets or light cloths. As the lifeguard first responder, pay particular attention to the injured guest's respiration and assist breathing if necessary.
3. Activate the Emergency Action System/EMS.

Third Degree Burns   Third degree burns damage all layers of the skin and can be multicolored (black, red, gray, white). These burns cause little or no pain in the third degree burn area. This phenomenon is a result of the destruction of local nerve endings. The patient will, however, suffer extreme pain in the areas around a third degree burn because of accompanying second degree burns.

Emergency Treatment for Third Degree Burns:

1. As the lifeguard first responder, your primary concern for injured guests with third degree burns should be to stop the burning process and simultaneously maintain an open airway. Look for signs of soot or burning around the face, mouth and nose.
2. After the airway is clear and breathing is adequate, you can then begin emergency care of the burn area.
3. All third degree burns should be covered with a clean dry cloth.
4. The lifeguard first responder should quickly remove all jewelry in the burn area and pay close attention to the injured guest's respirations.

All injured guests with third degree burns should be immediately transported to the hospital.

Chemical Burns

Chemical burns can cause all three degrees of burn damage. You must first take precautions to protect yourself from contact with the offending chemical. If the chemical is dry, quickly brush off the chemical using a cloth, broom, or newspaper. When you have removed most of the dry chemical, the area can be flushed with a lot of water for at least 15 minutes. If the chemical is in liquid form, begin flushing the area immediately.

Electrical Burns

Electrical burns can be very misleading for the lifeguard first responder. In many cases of electrocution, the real damage lies underneath the skin. For electrocuted guests, the lifeguard first responder must **ALWAYS** make sure the source of the electrocution has been removed. **Never assume the power source is off; always make sure before moving into the area.**

The external burns from electrocution can be treated similarly to thermal burns. However, the injured guest's external burns are usually only a small portion of the total tissue damage. The lifeguard first responder should focus on the ABC's and quickly activate the Emergency Action System/EMS.

Lightning

Victims of lightning electrocutions commonly suffer severe burns and are found pulseless and not breathing. Proper care begins as you immediately remove the injured guest from the area and begin a primary survey. Lifeguard first responders should begin CPR on those injured guests who have no obvious mortal wounds, even though they may look dead. Continue CPR until the EMS professionals arrive.

HEAT- AND COLD-RELATED EMERGENCIES

Objectives

- ◆ Recognize the causes of heat- and cold-related emergencies.
- ◆ Recognize the signs and symptoms of heat cramps, heat exhaustion, heat stroke, and hypothermia.
- ◆ Demonstrate the appropriate emergency treatment for heat cramps, heat exhaustion, heat stroke, and hypothermia.

As lifeguard first responders, you will most likely come in contact with guests who are suffering from heat-related problems. The injured guest's recovery will be directly related to your ability to recognize the different signs and symptoms of each type of heat emergency and render the appropriate care. You may also encounter guests who are suffering from cold-related problems, especially if the water is cold.

Heat Cramps

The guest suffering from heat cramps will complain of muscle cramps most commonly in the calf, muscle of the leg, and abdomen. The injured guest may also complain of dizziness, nausea/vomiting, and fatigue. The guest's skin will be hot and sweaty.

Emergency Treatment for Heat Cramps:

1. Move the guest to a cooler location and administer cool water (about 1/2 glass every 15 minutes). If cool water is not available, a diluted juice drink would work. Do not administer salt tablets. Salt makes many injured guests nauseated and may result in vomiting.
2. Activate the EMS/EAS if the patient does not improve quickly.

Heat Exhaustion

The guest suffering from heat exhaustion has lost significant amounts of fluid from perspiration. He or she will complain of a severe headache, nausea/vomiting, profuse sweating, fatigue, and even diarrhea. The skin will be cool, sweaty, and pale. The guest will be extremely thirsty.

Emergency Treatment for Heat Exhaustion:

1. Remove the injured guest from the heat source and begin to cool the injured guest.

2. Remove as much of the clothing as possible.

3. Elevate the guest's legs approximately 8 to 12 inches.

4. Administer cool water slowly and monitor the airway, watch for vomiting.

5. Activate the Emergency Action System/EMS if the injured guest does not improve.

Heat Stroke

Heat stroke is a **LIFE-THREATENING CONDITION** and requires immediate action by the lifeguard first responder to save the injured guest's life. The guest suffering from heat stroke will have extremely hot skin, which can be either wet or dry, a rapid pulse, tremors, mental confusion (including unconsciousness), nausea/vomiting, seizures, and snoring-like breathing.

Emergency Treatment for Heat Stroke:

1. Act rapidly in treating heat stroke as fast and aggressive cooling can make the difference between life or death. Seconds really do count here!

2. Establish an open airway initially and assist breathing as necessary. If CPR becomes necessary, this can be done while others rapidly cool the injured guest. Obviously, every guest with heat stroke should be removed from the heat source.

3. Remove all clothing as it traps in the heat.

4. Use whatever materials are available to cool the body. Ice packs in the armpits and groin work very well. Pour cool water over the body and vigorously fan the area. Do whatever is necessary to rapidly cool the injured guest. Use wrapped ice packs, or keep the guest wet by placing wet sheets or T-shirts over the guest and vigorously fan.

5. Continue cooling until the injured guest begins to shiver or is transported. Heat stroke can recur after cooling so watch the injured guest constantly.

Hypothermia

The lifeguard first responder is most likely to encounter hypothermia as a result of a guest staying in cold water long enough to begin to affect the core body temperature. If you recognize the beginning signs (shivering, numbness, blue lips) and symptoms of hypothermia in a guest, have them get out of the water and warm up.

Signs and Symptoms

◆ Shivering.

◆ Numbness.

◆ Blue lips.

◆ Inability to concentrate.

◆ Speech difficulty.

◆ Indifference.

◆ Decreased level of consciousness.

◆ Weakness/drowsiness.

If a guest has lost the ability to concentrate, you will need to take more aggressive measures to warm them. Place the guest in a warm shower until the symptoms begin to decrease. Follow with warm dry clothing. Warm beverages may be given if the guest is not unconscious.

Severe hypothermia is life-threatening, and requires special care when re-warming. Activate EMS if a guest is semi-conscious and monitor ABC's.

MUSCULOSKELETAL INJURIES

Objective

◆ Recognize and render emergency care for sprains, strains, dislocations, and fractures.

Signs and Symptoms

Musculoskeletal injuries in almost every case are not life-threatening. As the lifeguard first responder you must always first treat the primary A, B, C, and H and then render emergency care for the musculoskeletal problem. These musculoskeletal injuries share very similar signs and symptoms, and it can be very difficult or impossible to determine the exact type of problem you are treating. Remember your role as a lifeguard first responder is to provide care to keep further injury from occurring until EMS arrives.

Musculoskeletal injuries are divided into four categories: sprains, strains, dislocations, and fractures:

◆ **Sprains** involve the tearing of ligaments from muscle and cause local pain, local tenderness, increased pain with movement, and massive swelling.

◆ **Strains** involve the tearing of tendons or muscle and cause instant burning pain, very little swelling, and very little discoloration.

◆ **Dislocations** involve the displacement of bone joints. Dislocations usually cause obvious deformity, local pain, and loss of movement.

These particular injuries can appear very grotesque. The lifeguard first responder should remember, however, that all dislocations are treated after completing and controlling the primary survey.

- **Fractures** involve a break in the bone. Fractures are classified as either open or closed. In rare cases fractures can be life-threatening. The injured guest with a fracture will complain of pain, tenderness, swelling, bruising, and grating of bone ends. Exposed bone ends may even be seen.

Emergency Treatment for Musculoskeletal Injuries:

1. Remember that the majority of these injuries are non-life-threatening and a primary survey should be completed before caring for the musculoskeletal injury. The one exception is open fractures that include massive bleeding. This bleeding should be controlled under "H" of the primary survey.

2. Quickly expose the affected area and look for bruising, swelling, and bone ends. If the injured guest is unable to move the area, you should immediately splint the area.

3. Splinting can be accomplished using several items. You do not need a commercial splint to effectively stabilize the injured area.

4. You should not attempt to move the affected area; splint it in the position found. Always place the splint so that the joint above and the joint below the injury site cannot move. For example, if a guest has a forearm injury (you suspect a fracture) place a splint beyond the elbow and beyond the wrist.

5. The splint can be made using anything rigid and lightweight. The splint should also be long and wide enough to properly stabilize the injury. If you are unable to find a splint use the injured guest's body and bind the injured area to the body.

6. If the injured guest cannot move or has injured his or her head or neck, have the guest lay still, activate the Emergency Action System/EMS and maintain the A, B, C, and H.

7. If you do not suspect a possible fracture, splint the injured site, place a bag of ice over the affected area (protect by placing a cloth between the injured site and the ice), and elevate the site. After 20 minutes of ice apply a compression (Ace) bandage.

SOFT TISSUE INJURIES AND BLEEDING CONTROL

Objectives

- Describe the general types of soft tissue injuries including contusions, abrasions, lacerations, punctures, avulsions (skin flap), and amputations.

♦ Demonstrate the emergency care for soft tissue wounds, including proper care for amputations.

Soft tissue wounds are one of the most common injuries you will treat. These wounds are generally not life-threatening despite all the blood. The injuries can range from being as minor as a skinned knee (abrasion) to a major traumatic amputation. As a lifeguard first responder treating a soft tissue wound, you must be concerned with controlling bleeding and reducing the chances of infection. As with any situation where you might possibly come in contact with the injured guest's body fluids you must always use **Universal Precautions.**

Signs and Symptoms

♦ Most soft tissue wounds will have associated bleeding. This bleeding can be either internal (bruising) or external. If bleeding is external, you must quickly determine if the bleeding is coming from the arteries. Bleeding that is pumping ("squirting") comes from arteries and must be controlled immediately. Do not try to determine if the blood is "bright red," **IT DOES NOT MATTER, SINCE BLOOD IS BLOOD.** Arterial bleeding and severe veinous blood flow must be found and treated during the primary survey.

♦ Victims of soft tissue injuries can often have other associated injuries and be experiencing pain that does not fit the obvious wound. Remember to carefully conduct a secondary survey. Swelling is also common with soft tissue injuries that are causing internal bleeding.

Emergency Treatment for Soft Tissue Injuries:

1. Immediately complete the primary survey and determine if bleeding (hemorrhaging) is severe. If the bleeding is severe or significant, immediately apply direct pressure and elevate the wound above the level of the heart. Use a clean dry gauze pad or other clean material directly against the wound.

2. If the bleeding continues and the first gauze pad becomes soaked, apply additional gauze without removing the first.

3. In most cases this is all that will be necessary for the first several minutes. If bleeding continues, apply firm pressure over the main pressure points.

4. If bleeding continues, professional help is not available, and the injured guest is in danger of bleeding to death, consider a tourniquet.

5. **Never use a tourniquet unless professional help is not available, the other previous techniques have failed, and the person is going to bleed to death.**

A tourniquet can be made from material that is at least 2 inches wide and several inches long. A wide belt usually works well. Wrap the tourniquet around the limb (as close to the wound as possible) and tighten until the bleeding slows or stops.

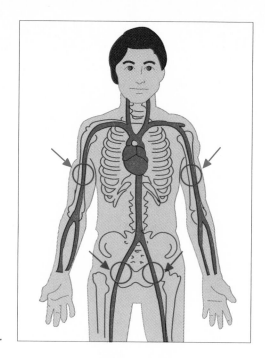

Pressure points.

Impaled Objects

If the soft tissue injury includes an impaled object, leave the object in place. The object should be stabilized until the EMS team arrives. The simplest method available to stabilize the impaled object is with both your hands or by packing a towel around it. Let the EMS professionals determine the best method of stabilization and transportation.

Amputations

If the soft tissue injury includes an amputated part, you must **First** complete a primary survey and then give emergency care for the amputated tissue:

1. Direct pressure should be applied to the stump and bleeding controlled. If this is all that you do prior to arrival of EMS, then you have been successful.

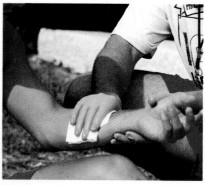

Direct pressure.

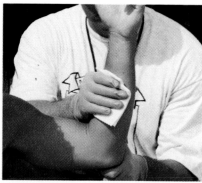

Elevation.

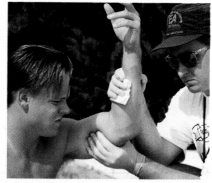

Direct pressure, elevation plus pressure point.

2. If time allows or bystanders are available, find the severed part. If found, place the part in a clean, moist cloth (gauze).

3. Place the wrapped part in a plastic bag and seal it.

4. Next, lay that plastic bag on top of a separate bag of ice. Make sure the part is not buried in ice or in direct contact with ice.

5. Transport the amputated part with the injured guest.

Nosebleeds

Nasal bleeding is a relatively common occurrence, especially in crowded conditions in an aquatic facility where the nose can be easily bumped or hit. The main objective should be to have the guest control the bleeding so that the lifeguard first responder does not come in contact with bodily fluids. Additionally, seek to minimize the amount of blood that goes down the guest's throat and into the stomach to reduce the chance of vomiting.

Emergency Treatment for Nosebleeds:

1. Seat the guest leaning slightly forward.

2. Have the guest pinch the nostrils together. If they are unable to do this, use Universal Precautions while you apply pressure by pinching the nostrils.

3. Hold the pinch for at least 5 minutes, and then gently release the nostrils to check if the bleeding has stopped.

4. If the bleeding has not stopped, repeat the pinch.

5. If the bleeding continues after an additional 5 minutes, seek medical attention.

FAINTING/SEIZURES

Objectives

◆ Understand the common causes of fainting.

◆ Recognize and treat the injured guest for fainting.

◆ Understand the possible causes of seizures.

◆ Demonstrate the appropriate emergency care for seizuring guests.

Fainting

Fainting occurs when the flow of blood containing oxygen to the brain is temporarily disrupted. Usually the guest will feel lightheaded and then quickly lose consciousness. Fainting guests will regain consciousness quickly after laying in a horizontal position. Some guests will have early warning signs/symptoms of an impending fainting episode. These signs/symptoms include nausea, weakness, chills, abdominal pain, or a pounding headache. Fainting is rarely serious and in most cases self-corrects after a few short moments. Causes of fainting include hyperventilation, hypoglycemia (low blood sugar), heart attacks, epilepsy, heart disease, dehydration, blood loss, or psychological stressors.

Emergency Treatment for Fainting:

1. If the guest has not fainted but complains of "feeling like fainting" quickly lay the guest down. This can prevent possible head and/or spinal injuries. Monitor the guest's ABC's.

2. If the guest has already fainted, look for signs of spinal injury and treat accordingly.

3. Monitor the guest's ABC's.

4. Look for any active bleeding.

5. Elevate the legs approximately 8 to 12 inches.

6. Watch for vomiting; if vomiting is possible, place the injured guest on his or her side in the recovery position.

7. Loosen any restrictive clothing.

8. Wipe forehead and face with cool, wet cloth.

Seizures

Seizures are sudden involuntary changes in the activity level of brain cells. These sudden changes can occur in sensation, behavior, muscle rigidity, or level of consciousness. Causes of seizures include epilepsy, infection, alcohol, trauma, stroke, overdose, tumors, fever, psychological stress, burns, or pregnancy.

Although there are many different causes of seizures, the lifeguard first responder should remember that the emergency treatment is very similar regardless of the cause. Millions of people suffer seizures each year, so be prepared to appropriately treat the seizuring guest.

Emergency Treatment for Seizures:

1. Immediately activate the EAS/EMS.

2. Carefully move any objects that may injure the guest.

3. Place a pillow or soft object between the guest's head and the floor.

4. Carefully maintain an open airway after the seizure subsides.

5. Complete the primary survey.

6. Take the necessary precautions if possible head/spinal injury has occurred.

7. Reassure the patient quietly and calmly as he or she regains consciousness.

8. Monitor the airway; be alert for vomiting.

9. Keep the guest warm.

10. Protect the guest's privacy.

11. Assist the guest out of the park.

   Never force anything into the mouth of a seizuring guest.

   Never attempt to restrain the seizuring guest.

   Never give the seizuring guest food or drink.

SHOCK

Objectives

◆ Recognize the signs and symptoms of three types of shock, including hypovolemic, anaphylactic, and insulin shock related to diabetic emergencies.

◆ Demonstrate the skills necessary to manage an injured guest exhibiting shock symptoms.

Shock is defined as a collapse of circulatory function caused by severe injury, blood loss, trauma, or disease. When shock occurs, oxygen is not being circulated to the vital organs such as the heart, lungs and brain. Untreated shock can be fatal. Another type of shock can also occur in people who have diabetes, and is related to an imbalance in the blood sugar level.

While there are several different types of shock, three are commonly treated by the lifeguard first responder. Hypovolemic shock occurs when too much blood is lost from the circulation system or following increased losses of body fluids. Anaphylactic shock occurs when the body has a very severe allergic reaction. Insulin shock is a condition related specifically to individuals who have diabetes. Each type of shock requires quick emergency care to stabilize the body and stop the shock process.

Hypovolemic Shock—Signs and Symptoms

◆ Breathing difficulties.

◆ Disorientation or confusion.

◆ Weak, rapid pulse.

◆ Nausea and vomiting.

◆ Extreme thirst.

◆ Cold, moist skin.

◆ Weakness.

Emergency Treatment for Hypovolemic Shock:

1. Immediately complete and control the A, B, C, and H.
2. Activate the EAS/EMS.
3. Pay particular attention to all bleeding wounds and check for signs of internal bleeding such as bruising or tenderness.
4. Preserve body heat, but **do not overheat.**
5. If the guest is conscious and does not have a suspected spinal injury, elevate the legs approximately 8–12 inches.
6. If the guest is unconscious and does not have a suspected spinal injury, place them on their side in the recovery position and watch for vomiting.
7. Monitor the A, B, C, and H.

Anaphylactic Shock—Signs and Symptoms

- Respiratory wheezes.
- Squeezing sensation in the chest.
- Swelling in the airway.
- Weak, rapid pulse.
- Massive swelling.
- Blueness around the mouth and lips.
- Itching and burning of the skin.
- Hives.

Emergency Treatment for Anaphylactic Shock:

1. Immediately complete and control the A, B, C, and H. Initiate CPR if needed.
2. Do not be fooled by minor signs of distress. Anaphylactic shock can occur within seconds!
3. Activate the EAS/EMS.
4. Maintain the airway, assist breathing as needed.
5. If allergic reaction is from a bee sting, find the stinger location and scrape the stinger off. **Do not pluck out the stinger.** If you pinch the top of the stinger you may inject more bee venom into the guest.
6. Determine if the guest has medication for allergic reactions and help them self-administer their medicine. If they are unable to self-administer, follow directions on the kit.

Lifeguard first responders must not forget that anaphylactic shock is a life-threatening condition. Immediate intervention is necessary to save the injured guest's life. If the injured guest complains even of slight discomfort, quickly activate the Emergency Action System/EMS and treat accordingly.

DIABETIC EMERGENCIES

A person with diabetes must regulate their levels of blood sugar and insulin with medication, diet, and exercise. Keeping this condition under control can sometimes be difficult, and an imbalance of either sugar or insulin can result in two types of emergencies that require immediate care.

Insulin shock (hypoglycemia) occurs when the level of insulin is too high, and the level of blood sugar is too low. The symptoms can develop rapidly, and can be caused by a person with diabetes taking too much of their medication, not eating at regular intervals, or exercising heavily. A person in insulin shock needs to quickly get sugar into the blood to counteract the high level of insulin.

Diabetic coma (hyperglycemia) occurs when the level of blood sugar is too high and the level of insulin is too low. The symptoms usually develop slowly over a few days.

Insulin Shock—Signs and Symptoms

- Rapid pulse.
- Fast breathing.
- Sweating.
- Weakness.
- Hunger.
- Vision difficulties.
- Change in level of consciousness.
- Numbness in hands and feet.

Emergency Treatment for Insulin Shock:

1. If the guest is conscious, they may often know what to do and can direct you, and may be able to help you determine when they have eaten or taken their medication. Give the conscious guest anything that contains sugar such as juice or a fruit drink, candy, or soft drink.
2. Monitor A, B, C's until symptoms subside.
3. If a guest is unconscious, activate EAS/EMS. Place a small amount of sugar under their tongue (no liquids).
4. Place guest in recovery position and watch for vomiting.

Diabetic Coma—Signs and Symptoms

- Drowsiness.
- Confusion.
- Fever.
- Thirst.

◆ Deep, fast breathing.

◆ Change in level of consciousness.

◆ Fruity breath odor.

Emergency Treatment for Diabetic Coma:

1. Activate EAS/EMS.

2. Monitor the A, B, C's.

If you are unsure during a diabetic emergency that a conscious guest is suffering is insulin shock or the beginning stages of a diabetic coma, treat it as if it is insulin shock by immediately giving sugar. Symptoms will rapidly subside if it is insulin shock, and the emergency will be successfully managed. Sugar will not cause further harm or reduce symptoms of diabetic coma.

ASTHMA EMERGENCIES

Objectives

◆ Recognize the signs and symptoms of a guest experiencing an asthma attack.

◆ Demonstrate the skills necessary to manage a guest experiencing an asthma attack.

Asthma is a chronic (ongoing) condition that causes periods of difficult breathing. When a person experiences an attack, the passageways to the lungs narrow, tissues lining the passages constrict and are blocked with mucus. Breathing becomes difficult and usually needs to be controlled with medication.

Asthma attacks can be brought on by many things, including infections, exercise, allergies, and sensitivity to drugs and chemicals. Most people know they have asthma and are used to dealing with an attack, but many people are unaware of their condition and a first attack may take them by surprise.

A severe or prolonged asthma attack that does not respond to aggressive treatment is life-threatening and requires immediate medical attention.

Asthma—Signs and Symptoms

◆ Fighting for breath.

◆ Spasmodic coughing.

◆ Whistling or high-pitched wheezing.

◆ Rapid, shallow breaths.

◆ Fatigue.

◆ Stomach cramps, especially in young children.

Emergency Treatment for Asthma

1. Help the injured guest to a straight up sitting position.

2. Assist the injured guest in using an inhaler if they have their medication with them.

3. Monitor ABC's and activate EAS/EMS if symptoms do not get better.

POISONING EMERGENCIES

Objectives

◆ Recognize the signs and symptoms of inhaled and swallowed poisoning.

◆ Demonstrate the skills necessary to manage a poisoning emergency.

A poison is any substance—liquid, solid or gas that impairs health or causes death by its chemical action when it is introduced into the body or onto the skin surfaces. Poisons may enter the body by ingestion, inhalation, injection or absorption.

The signs and symptoms of poisoning vary according to the substances involved. In the case of any poisoning emergency, you will need to contact your regional poison control center as part of your EAS/EAP. Also remember that you should always protect **yourself** first when dealing with poison emergencies.

Inhaled Poison—Signs and Symptoms

◆ Severe headache.

◆ Nausea and/or vomiting.

◆ Facial burns.

◆ Burning sensation in throat or chest.

◆ Discoloration of the lips.

◆ Difficulty breathing.

◆ Coughing.

◆ Altered levels of consciousness.

◆ Dizziness.

Emergency Treatment for Inhaled Poison:

1. Activate EAS/EMS.

2. Protect yourself. Remove guest from source to fresh air.

3. Monitor the ABC's and perform rescue breathing and CPR as needed.

Swallowed Poison—Signs and Symptoms

- ◆ Nausea.
- ◆ Vomiting.
- ◆ Diarrhea.
- ◆ Drowsiness.
- ◆ Abnormal breathing.
- ◆ Unusual breath or body odor.
- ◆ Convulsions.
- ◆ Burns around the mouth.

Emergency Treatment for Swallowed Poison:

1. Activate EAS/EMS.
2. Monitor ABC's and treat accordingly.
3. Contact regional poison control center, try to identify what and how much was ingested.
4. Follow instructions from poison control center related to inducing vomiting or other emergency care.
5. Continue to monitor ABC's until EMS arrives.

KEY CONCEPTS IN LIFEGUARD FIRST RESPONDER EMERGENCY CARE

- ◆ Lifeguard first responders are not a replacement of the Emergency Action System/EMS professionals; activate the Emergency Action System/EMS early.
- ◆ Lifeguard first responders must be primarily concerned with their own safety in every rescue/emergency situation.
- ◆ Every injured guest must first receive a complete primary survey (A, B, C, and H).
- ◆ **Problems found in the primary survey must be controlled before all other problems. NO exceptions!**
- ◆ A secondary survey begins at the head and ends at the toes. The lifeguard first responder must complete this survey only after the primary A, B, C, and H are controlled. This survey is completed by touching, looking and asking.
- ◆ Maintain spinal cord stabilization in all guests suspected of having a serious head injury.
- ◆ Follow local emergency care protocols if they differ from what you have learned.
- ◆ Practice all emergency care skills constantly.

- Document your emergency treatment immediately.
- After emergency care has been completed and properly documented, return to your assigned zone.

REVIEW QUESTIONS

1. T F   Basic first responder skills, if not performed, could lead to additional injury and possible death for the guest.

2. T F   Life-threatening emergencies for the lifeguard first responder are those that compromise the guest's airway, breathing, or circulation in any manner, including those situations in which massive bleeding is found.

3. T F   As a lifeguard first responder, your safety comes second.

4. T F   Guests cannot be breathing but still have a pulse.

5. T F   Guests without a pulse will not be breathing.

6. When do you perform a secondary survey?

   _____

7. What are you looking for in a secondary survey, and what do you do with the information? _____

8. Match the symptoms with the type of burn:

   _____ First degree   a. Blisters, extreme pain
   _____ Second degree   b. No pain at actual burn area, multicolored skin
   _____ Third degree   c. Red skin, slight swelling, pain

9. Match the type of burn with emergency treatment:

   _____ First degree   a. Place area in cool water until pain stops

   _____ Second degree   b. Maintain airway, cover with clean cloth, transport to hospital

   _____ Third degree   c. Cover area with moist, clean sheets

10. In addition to heat or flame, list three other sources of burns and how to treat them:

    a.
    b.
    c.

11. Match the symptoms with the type of heat emergency:

    _____ Heat cramps   a. Hot skin, rapid pulse, tremors, confusion

    _____ Heat exhaustion   b. Cool, sweaty, pale skin; nausea, headache

    _____ Heat stroke   c. Leg, abdomen, calf cramps plus dizziness; nausea

12. T F   Heat stroke is a life-threatening condition.

13. T F   Sprains, strains, dislocations, and fractures should be cared for only after doing a primary survey and finding everything OK.

14. T F   Bleeding that is "squirting" comes from arteries, and must be controlled immediately.

15. Matching:

_____ Direct pressure	a. Skin flap injury
_____ Elevation	b. Bruise
_____ Pressure points	c. Scrape
_____ Contusion	d. First method of controlling bleeding
_____ Abrasion	e. Protecting yourself from contact with body fluids
_____ Avulsion	f. Along with direct pressure, the second stage of controlling bleeding
_____ Universal Precautions	g. Places around the body where an artery can be pressed against bone to slow the flow of blood

16. T F   To treat fainting without head or neck injury, monitor the guest's ABC's, look for any active bleeding, elevate legs, loosen restrictive clothing, and place in recovery position until the guest feels better.

17. T F   There are many different causes of seizures, and each must be treated differently.

18. T F   Never force anything into the mouth of a seizuring guest, attempt to restrain him or her, or give food or drink.

19. The type of shock that occurs when the body has a severe allergic reaction is called _____ .

20. If a guest has been stung or bitten by an insect and is exhibiting signs of a reaction, you should activate EAS/EMS and find out if the guest has any _____ to control the reaction.

21. When treating a soft tissue wound, your role as a lifeguard first responder is to

    a.

    b.

22. T F   When treating for hypovolemic shock, keep the guest warm, with elevated legs, but do not overheat.

23. T F   Lifeguard first responders are not a replacement for the EAS/EMS professionals—activate the EAS/EMS early.

SKILL SHEET 13

Head, Eye, and Dental Emergencies

■ HEAD INJURIES ■

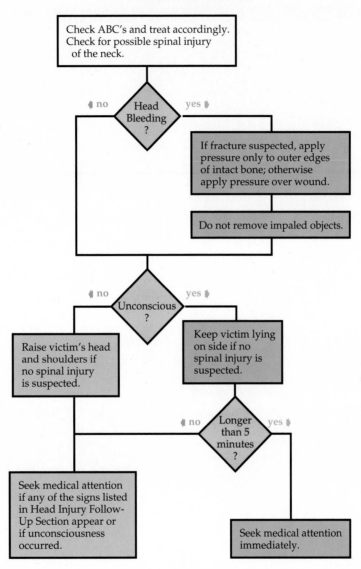

Head, Eye, and Dental Emergencies
▦ DENTAL INJURIES ▦

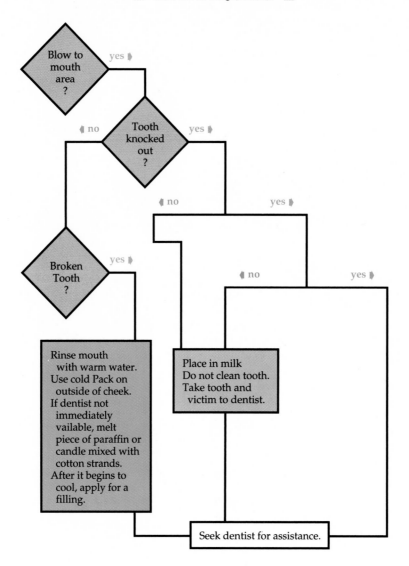

Blow to mouth area ? — yes ▶

◀ no — **Tooth knocked out ?** — yes ▶

◀ no   yes ▶

Broken Tooth ? — yes ▶

◀ no   yes ▶

Rinse mouth with warm water. Use cold Pack on outside of cheek. If dentist not immediately vailable, melt piece of paraffin or candle mixed with cotton strands. After it begins to cool, apply for a filling.

Place in milk
Do not clean tooth.
Take tooth and victim to dentist.

Seek dentist for assistance.

Head, Eye, and Dental Emergencies

▨ EYE INJURIES ▨

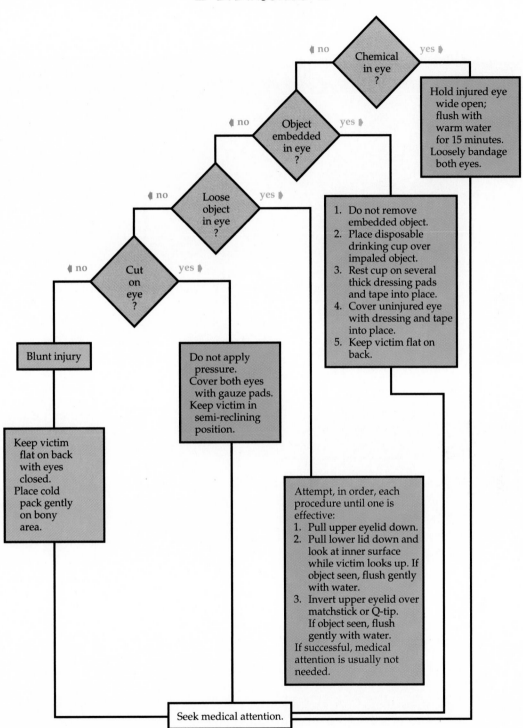

Chemical in eye ?
‹ no
yes ›

Hold injured eye wide open; flush with warm water for 15 minutes. Loosely bandage both eyes.

Object embedded in eye ?
‹ no
yes ›

Loose object in eye ?
‹ no
yes ›

1. Do not remove embedded object.
2. Place disposable drinking cup over impaled object.
3. Rest cup on several thick dressing pads and tape into place.
4. Cover uninjured eye with dressing and tape into place.
5. Keep victim flat on back.

Cut on eye ?
‹ no
yes ›

Blunt injury

Do not apply pressure. Cover both eyes with gauze pads. Keep victim in semi-reclining position.

Keep victim flat on back with eyes closed. Place cold pack gently on bony area.

Attempt, in order, each procedure until one is effective:
1. Pull upper eyelid down.
2. Pull lower lid down and look at inner surface while victim looks up. If object seen, flush gently with water.
3. Invert upper eyelid over matchstick or Q-tip. If object seen, flush gently with water.
If successful, medical attention is usually not needed.

Seek medical attention.

SKILL SHEET 14

Burn Emergencies

▨ HEAT BURNS (THERMAL) ▨

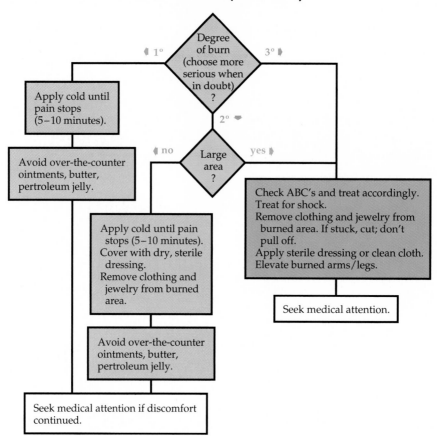

Burn Emergencies

ELECTRICAL INJURIES

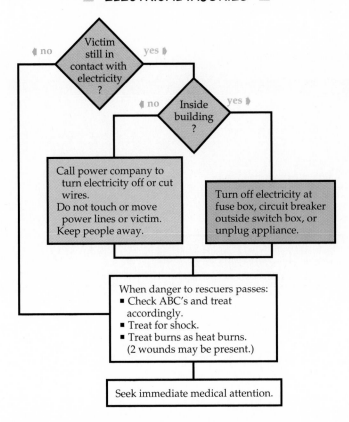

Victim still in contact with electricity?
- no
- yes

Inside building?
- no
- yes

Call power company to turn electricity off or cut wires.
Do not touch or move power lines or victim.
Keep people away.

Turn off electricity at fuse box, circuit breaker outside switch box, or unplug appliance.

When danger to rescuers passes:
- Check ABC's and treat accordingly.
- Treat for shock.
- Treat burns as heat burns. (2 wounds may be present.)

Seek immediate medical attention.

CHEMICAL BURNS

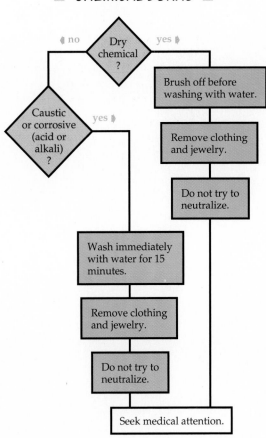

Dry chemical?
- no
- yes

Caustic or corrosive (acid or alkali)?
- yes

Brush off before washing with water.

Remove clothing and jewelry.

Do not try to neutralize.

Wash immediately with water for 15 minutes.

Remove clothing and jewelry.

Do not try to neutralize.

Seek medical attention.

SKILL SHEET 15

Temperature-Related Emergencies
▨ HEAT-RELATED EMERGENCIES ▨

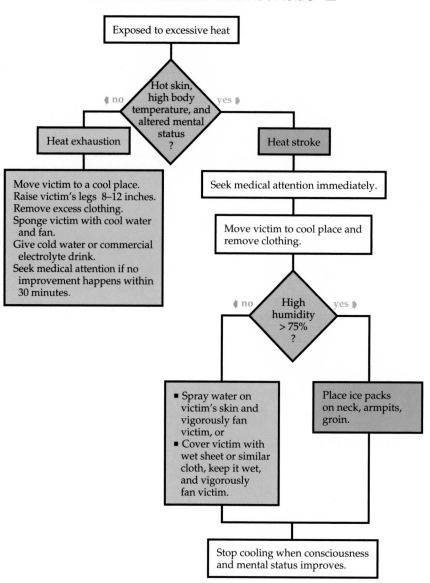

Temperature-Related Emergencies

▨ HYPOTHERMIA ▨

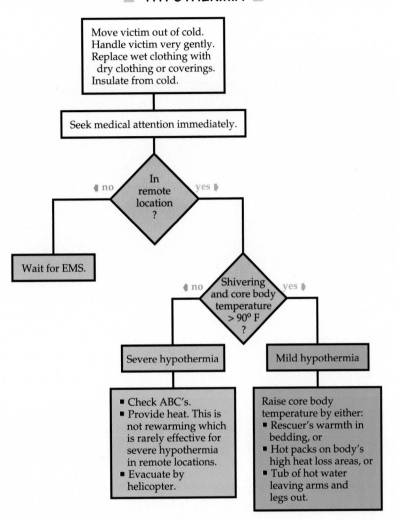

SKILL SHEET 16

Musculoskeletal Injury Emergencies

■ SPRAINS, STRAINS, CONTUSIONS, DISLOCATIONS ■

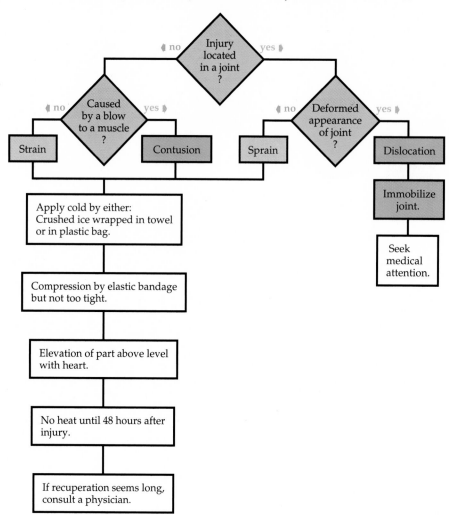

Musculoskeletal Injury Emergencies

▨ FRACTURES ▨

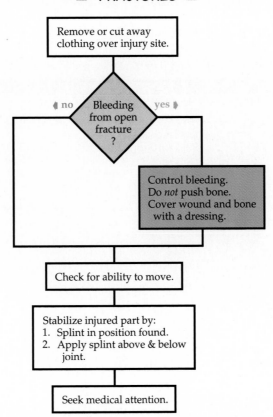

SKILL SHEET 17

Soft Tissue Injuries and Bleeding

▓ BLEEDING ▓

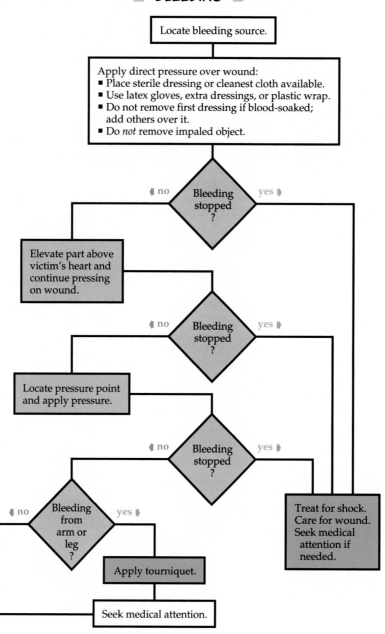

Locate bleeding source.

Apply direct pressure over wound:
- Place sterile dressing or cleanest cloth available.
- Use latex gloves, extra dressings, or plastic wrap.
- Do not remove first dressing if blood-soaked; add others over it.
- Do *not* remove impaled object.

Bleeding stopped?
— no → Elevate part above victim's heart and continue pressing on wound.
— yes → Treat for shock. Care for wound. Seek medical attention if needed.

Bleeding stopped?
— no → Locate pressure point and apply pressure.
— yes → Treat for shock. Care for wound. Seek medical attention if needed.

Bleeding stopped?
— no → Bleeding from arm or leg?
— yes → Treat for shock. Care for wound. Seek medical attention if needed.

Bleeding from arm or leg?
— no → Seek medical attention.
— yes → Apply tourniquet. → Seek medical attention.

Soft Tissue Injuries and Bleeding

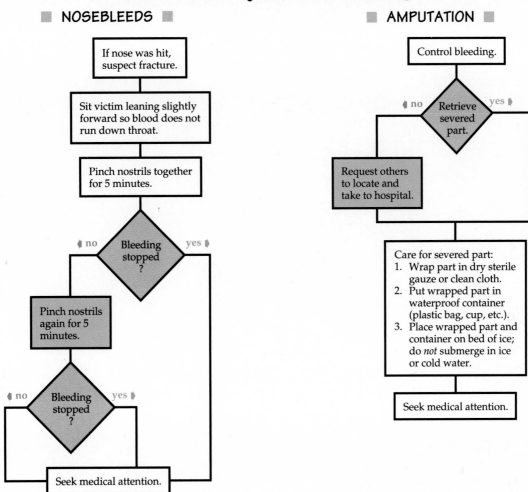

▨ NOSEBLEEDS ▨

If nose was hit, suspect fracture.

Sit victim leaning slightly forward so blood does not run down throat.

Pinch nostrils together for 5 minutes.

Bleeding stopped?
◄ no   yes ►

Pinch nostrils again for 5 minutes.

Bleeding stopped?
◄ no   yes ►

Seek medical attention.

▨ AMPUTATION ▨

Control bleeding.

Retrieve severed part.
◄ no   yes ►

Request others to locate and take to hospital.

Care for severed part:
1. Wrap part in dry sterile gauze or clean cloth.
2. Put wrapped part in waterproof container (plastic bag, cup, etc.).
3. Place wrapped part and container on bed of ice; do *not* submerge in ice or cold water.

Seek medical attention.

SKILL SHEET 18

Fainting and Seizure Emergencies

▨ FAINTING ▨

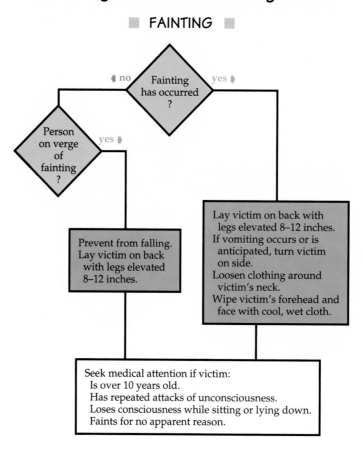

Fainting has occurred?
— no →
— yes →

Person on verge of fainting?
— yes →

Prevent from falling. Lay victim on back with legs elevated 8–12 inches.

Lay victim on back with legs elevated 8–12 inches.
If vomiting occurs or is anticipated, turn victim on side.
Loosen clothing around victim's neck.
Wipe victim's forehead and face with cool, wet cloth.

Seek medical attention if victim:
Is over 10 years old.
Has repeated attacks of unconsciousness.
Loses consciousness while sitting or lying down.
Faints for no apparent reason.

Fainting and Seizure Emergencies

■ SEIZURES ■

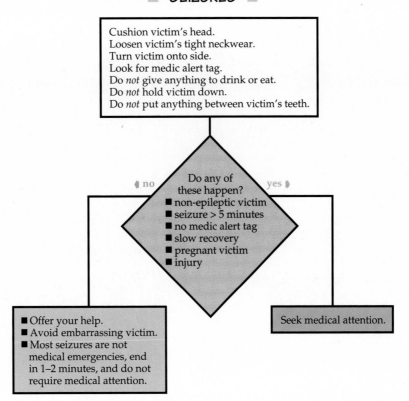

Cushion victim's head.
Loosen victim's tight neckwear.
Turn victim onto side.
Look for medic alert tag.
Do *not* give anything to drink or eat.
Do *not* hold victim down.
Do *not* put anything between victim's teeth.

Do any of
these happen?
■ non-epileptic victim
■ seizure > 5 minutes
■ no medic alert tag
■ slow recovery
■ pregnant victim
■ injury

◄ no   yes ►

■ Offer your help.
■ Avoid embarrassing victim.
■ Most seizures are not
medical emergencies, end
in 1–2 minutes, and do not
require medical attention.

Seek medical attention.

SKILL SHEET 19

Diabetic and Shock Emergencies

▨ **HYPOVOLEMIC SHOCK** ▨   ▨ **SEVERE ALLERGIC REACTION** ▨
                                        (Anaphylactic Shock)

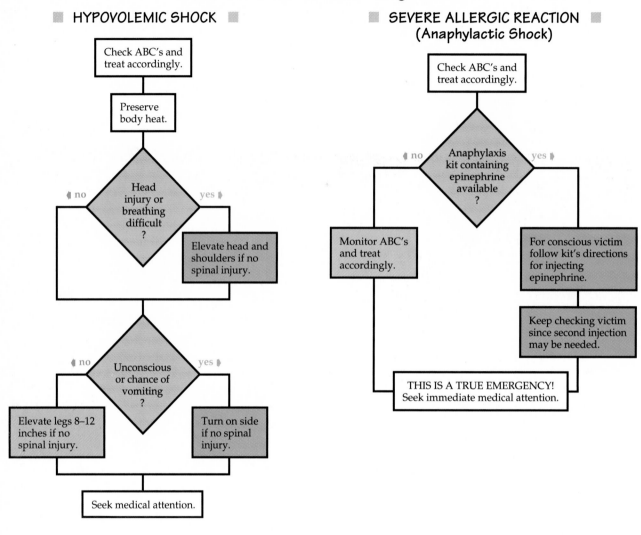

Diabetic and Shock Emergencies

▨ DIABETIC EMERGENCIES ▨

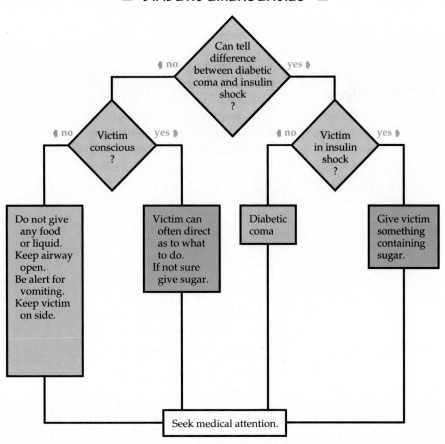

SKILL SHEET 20

Asthma and Poison Emergencies

▦ ASTHMA ▦

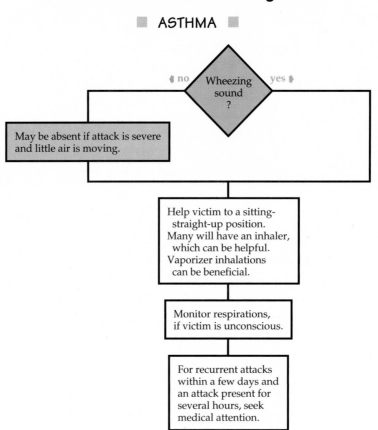

May be absent if attack is severe and little air is moving.

no ◀ **Wheezing sound ?** ▶ yes

Help victim to a sitting-straight-up position. Many will have an inhaler, which can be helpful. Vaporizer inhalations can be beneficial.

Monitor respirations, if victim is unconscious.

For recurrent attacks within a few days and an attack present for several hours, seek medical attention.

Asthma and Poison Emergencies

▨ INHALED POISON ▨

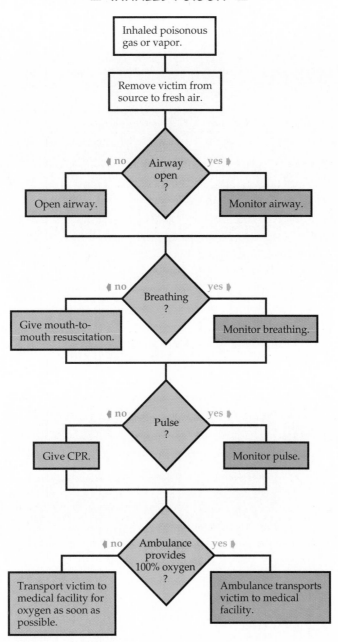

Asthma and Poison Emergencies
▨ SWALLOWED POISON ▨

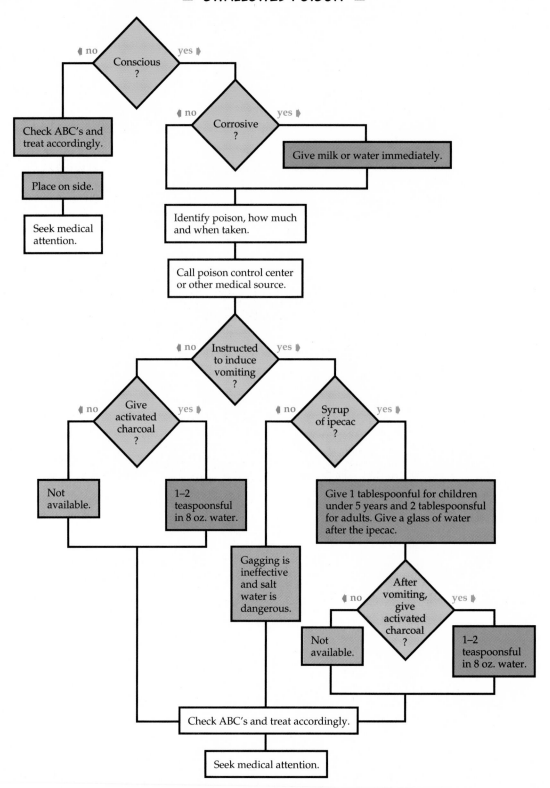

Professionalism

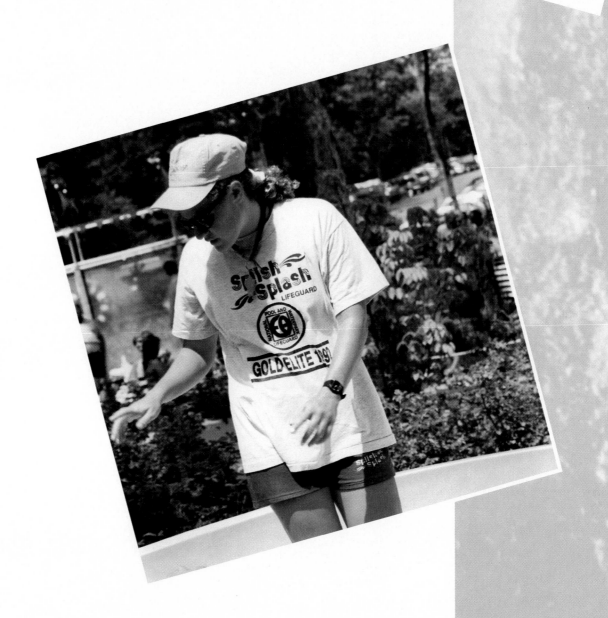

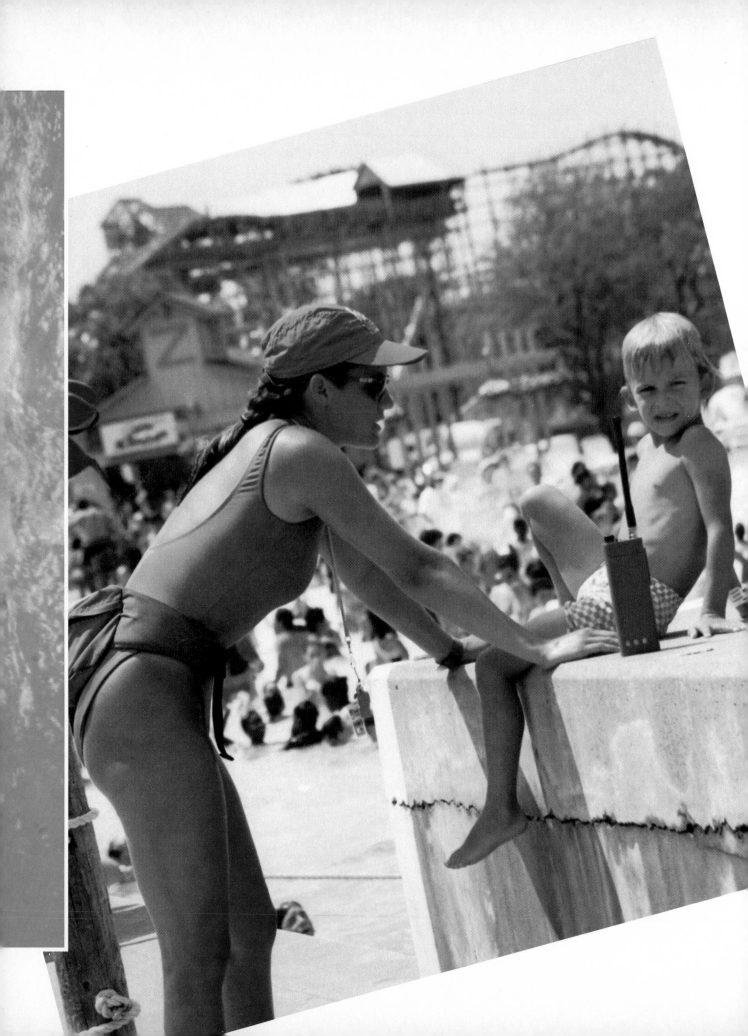

What Other Responsibilities Will I Have as a Lifeguard?

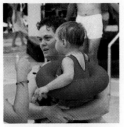

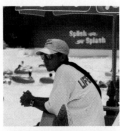

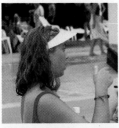

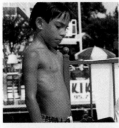

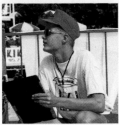

CHAPTER OBJECTIVES

After completing the chapter and related water work, the lifeguard candidate should be able to:

1. Identify at least four behaviors that help create a professional image.
2. Understand the key to good guest relations.
3. Identify four strategies for crowd control.
4. Understand the importance of paperwork and performing related duties.
5. Understand the importance of maintaining skill level.

As a lifeguard, your main responsibility is to prevent drownings. One aspect of this responsibility consists of managing people, controlling their actions, and providing for their health and safety.

PROFESSIONAL IMAGE

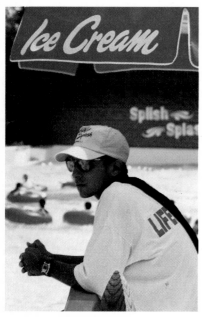

Project a professional image.

One of the key components of managing people is preparing yourself to be viewed as a professional. As a lifeguard, you are a very important part of the facility's team. You contribute to the whole environment: if you look and act like a professional, the facility looks like a well-run facility. Guests at the facility will constantly watch you; you are continually "on stage." If they view you as a professional, they will respond to your requests and directions much easier than if they do not have any respect for you or your position. To maintain your professional image:

- ◆ Arrive ahead of time.
- ◆ Be in full uniform, easily identified as a lifeguard, neat, and clean.
- ◆ Bring auxiliary items you need (whistle, sunscreen, etc.); be prepared.
- ◆ Be pleasant to staff and guests at all times.
- ◆ Pay attention to placement and condition of your rescue equipment.
- ◆ Perform your job well.

Guest Relations

It is part of your responsibility to make the guests who visit your facility feel welcome. Base all of your actions on the Golden Rule: **Treat people like you would like to be treated.**

You must also develop a sensitivity to people of diverse cultures who visit your facility. You should be open to ideas and input of guests and colleagues from various cultures and avoid being biased or judging others by their background.

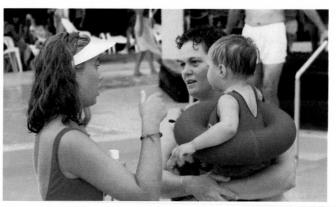

Remember the Golden Rule.

Remember also that dealing with people, including the public and co-workers and supervisors, becomes easier with experience. There are also many styles and approaches to people management that are equally effective. You must use a style and approach that suit your personality and scope of responsibility.

RULE ENFORCEMENT

Rule enforcement is always difficult. No one likes to have his or her actions restricted. Just as society is governed by laws, swimmers are governed by rules for their health and safety. Some rules will be enforced at **all** aquatic facilities, such as "No Running" or "No Glass On Deck." However, each facility will also have its own rules, and you must know the rules of your specific facility.

Understand and Explain the Rules

As a lifeguard, you should also understand the reason for a rule and be able to explain it. You may find that once you explain a rule to a swimmer, enforcing it will be very easy. Your goal is to prevent drownings, accidents, and injuries. If swimmers understand why certain actions are unsafe, they are less likely to repeat them. For example, replacing "Mister, you can't bring that bottle in here," with "I'm sorry sir, bottles are not allowed in the pool by order of the health department; broken glass in the pool is almost impossible to find and remove," is much more effective and positive.

Be Consistent in Enforcing Rules

To be consistent means to enforce the same rule in the same way every time. If you whistle at swimmers for some action today, you should whistle at them for the same action tomorrow.

Enforce Rules Uniformly

Uniform rule enforcement means that if two different swimmers are violating a rule, both should be stopped. Remember that rules should be fair for everyone using the pool.

Use the Positive Approach

When you make corrections, use the positive approach. For example, instead of saying "Don't run," say "Please walk." Remember that people swim for enjoyment and fun. We want them to be safe, but to also have a good time. As a professional lifeguard, the manner in which you enforce rules is very important.

Know Where the Rules Are Posted

It is a good idea to remind swimmers where the rules are posted. The posted rules are backup authority for you.

Refer Problems to Your Supervisor

If children keep violating a rule, have them sit out for a few minutes. Sometimes a time-out will solve a problem. If the problem persists, or if an older swimmer argues with you about a rule, do not hesitate to seek assistance from your supervisor. You cannot allow yourself to be distracted from your zone by spending a lot of time dealing with a guest. Whether that supervisor is the head lifeguard, assistant manager, or manager, a part of his or her job is to help you with rule enforcement. If there is any situation you cannot handle, get the help of your supervisor.

CROWD CONTROL

Situations may arise while you are on duty that would require you to control large numbers of guests and maintain order. Some examples would be a weather emergency or any emergency in which groups of people need to be moved or directed. Practicing your Emergency Action Plan will help you prepare for such an incident. If you need to control a crowd:

- Keep yourself calm.
- Speak loudly and clearly.
- Give precise, simple directions.
- Speak with authority.

PAPERWORK

Another responsibility you will have as a lifeguard is completing reports and maintaining records. Some examples of the types of recordkeeping you may have to be responsible for are: attendance, sign-in, maintenance schedule, pool chemistry, weather conditions, and documentation of in-service training.

The most important items of paperwork you will complete are the accident report and the rescue report. Each **rescue** requires careful documentation as soon as it has occurred. Use the report forms supplied by your facility and fill in each section completely. Following through on paperwork is another way of doing your job well and being a professional lifeguard.

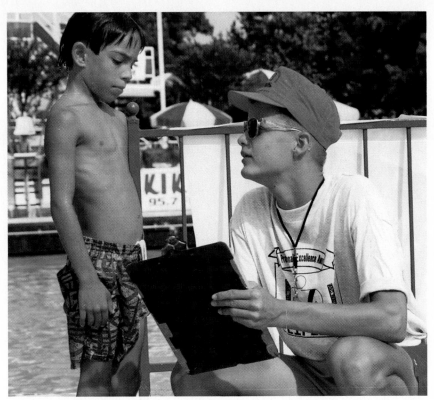

Follow through on paperwork.

RELATED DUTIES

Aquatic facilities often require their lifeguards to perform duties not directly related to the two primary responsibilities of preventing drownings/accidents and providing rescue and emergency care. These duties will vary depending upon the facility. It is the responsibility of your employer to provide you with a complete job description. Read the job description carefully so that you clearly understand your duties and responsibilities before beginning work.

MAINTAINING YOUR SKILLS

As a National Pool and Waterpark Lifeguard, you are responsible for maintaining your skills at "test ready" levels at all times. The skills you learn in this class will require constant review and practice. The in-service training you will participate in at your facility will help you maintain your skill level, but it is up to you to be sure that all of your observational, CPR, and technical rescue skills are reviewed regularly.

REVIEW QUESTIONS

1. Being professional means:
   a. Being in full uniform, easily identified and neat and clean.
   b. Being pleasant to guests and staff at all times.
   c. Paying attention to placement and condition of your rescue equipment.
   d. only (a) and (b).
   e. (a), (b), and (c).

2. List three things that might lessen the number of times you have to enforce a rule.
   a.
   b.
   c.

3. What is the Golden Rule?

   _____

4. List three things that will help you control a crowd.
   a.
   b.
   c.

5. T   F   Only rescues that involved CPR need documentation.

6. Working as a lifeguard means that you:
   a. Should expect to have regular in-service training.
   b. Could be physically injured.
   c. Might have to work in bad weather conditions.
   d. Might have to perform unrelated duties at your facility.
   e. Will be expected to maintain professional standards.
   f. All of the above.

SKILL SHEET 21

Lifeguard Responsibilities

1

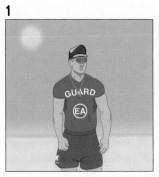

Professional image.

2

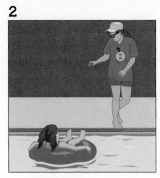

Guest relations.

3

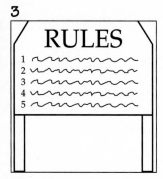

Rule enforcement.

4

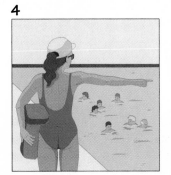

Crowd control.

5

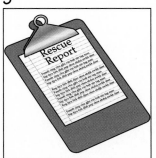

Paperwork.

6

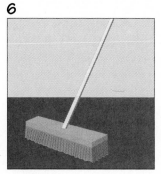

Related duties.

7

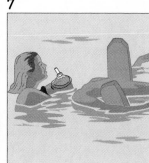

Maintain skill level.

KEY POINTS:

◆ Be courteous and kind to guests and fellow staff.

◆ Remember the Golden Rule.

◆ You can make a difference and save lives.

CRITICAL THINKING:

1. How would you handle an irate guest?

2. What is the best way to enforce a rule?

3. What types of nonlifeguarding related duties do you think you may have to do?

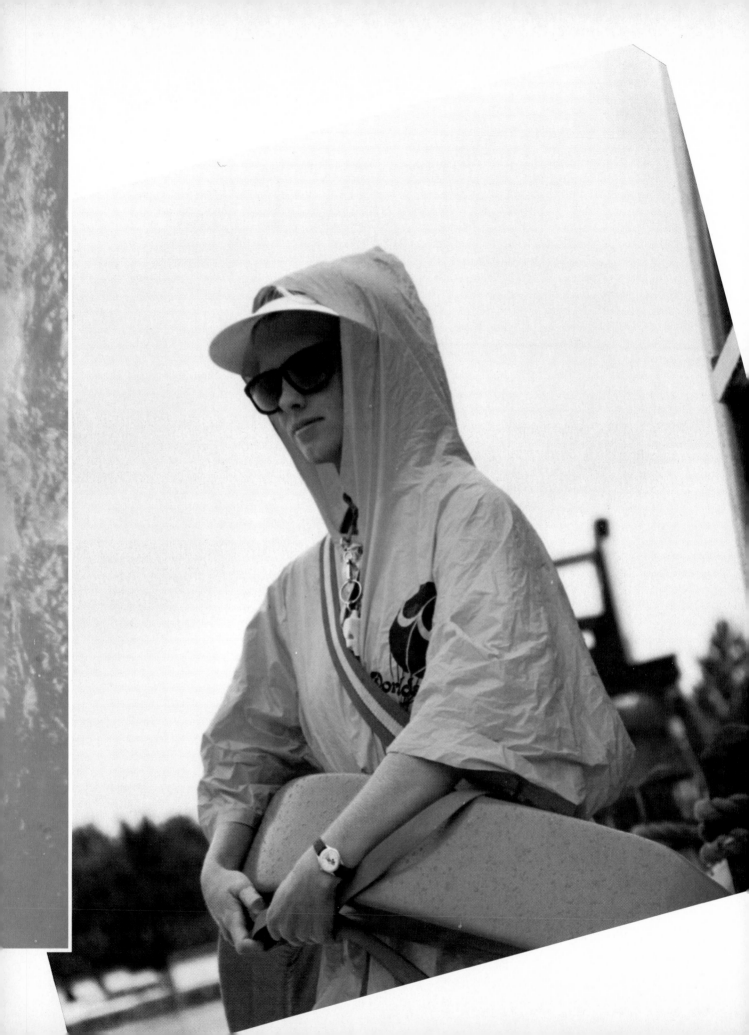

How Do I Adapt My Skills to Special Situations and Different Facilities?

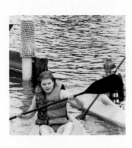

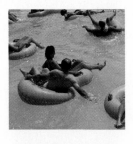

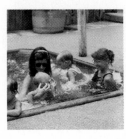

CHAPTER OBJECTIVES

After completing the chapter and related water work, the lifeguard candidate should be able to:

1. Understand the importance of adapting skills to the situation.
2. Identify strategies for lifeguarding the disabled.
3. Identify strategies for lifeguarding waterparks or special facilities.
4. Identify strategies for lifeguarding pools.
5. Identify strategies for lifeguarding special events.
6. Identify strategies for lifeguarding protected lakefronts.

Your primary responsibilities as a lifeguard will always remain the same, but situations may vary according to the type of facility, number of guests, type of guests, and nature of the aquatic attractions. Each of these situations will require you to adapt your skills to meet the needs of the moment.

LIFEGUARDING THE DISABLED PERSON

Since it is likely that there will be disabled persons swimming sometime at the facility where you lifeguard, there are some basic things you should know. First, and most important, is the fact that disabled persons are not different, in their likes and dislikes, from you or from anyone else. They like the water; they like the sun.

However, some *physically disabled* persons, because of their disability, may move differently: they may have balance problems or may not be able to control arm and leg movements as well as others. Some persons with *mental impairments* may not understand as rapidly as others when you explain rules. Some people with *sensory impairments* (hearing or vision) may communicate differently (or may need *you* to communicate differently). If you have knowledge about some of these differences in movement ability and understanding you can better meet the safety needs of these guests.

Movement Ability Differences

Some persons with a physical disability have difficulty with balance, and many will have less buoyancy and movement capacity. Many things can cause these differences:

◆ An individual with a leg missing may have difficulty with a balanced float, because the body will tend to roll (away from the side that has the leg missing). That person has to apply "counter balance"; they must learn to counteract the roll tendency by turning the head or moving the arms out to the side.

◆ Individuals whose legs are paralyzed may experience increased "drag" from those legs and may have to change the force or direction of arm pull, when they swim, to compensate. They also *will not be able to jump or catch themselves with their legs:* skills that are especially important in wave pools.

◆ Persons who have cerebral palsy may have less range of movement of arms or legs. They may not be able to reach as far or step as far. They might also have what are called "purposeless movements," when their arms and legs may move in ways the person doesn't direct them to. They, too, may have difficulties in a wave pool because of having less effective movement.

Communication Difficulties

Mentally retarded persons can learn, but may learn more slowly than most other people. If mentally retarded persons come to your facility, you may need to repeat some of the safety rules or remind them several times about the same thing. You need to keep your explanations short and simple. It is probably best if mentally retarded persons wear life-jackets, the first few times they are in a wave pool.

Persons with hearing or vision loss may communicate differently. If one of your senses doesn't work well, you tend to use the other senses more. Thus, blind persons *rely more on their hearing*, and deaf people *rely more on their vision.* You may have to communicate differently to persons with these disabilities:

◆ **Someone with a speech difficulty** might use sign language, writing, a symbol board, or even an interpreter to talk with you.

◆ If someone is trying to ask you a question, be sure that you find a way to understand this person, because the question could be critical.

◆ Be an assertive listener: give feedback and request feedback from the person, to find the level of understanding.

◆ **Visually impaired people** may need more specific instructions to orient them to the facility. Mention landmarks and "sound marks": sounds that are specific to a given area of the facility. Mention emergency sounds with specific reactions that are necessary.

◆ Give a verbal warning before you touch someone with a visual impairment.

◆ Do not use vague words when giving instructions—be specific. Try to give the person enough information so that they can use the facility independently with minimal help.

◆ **Someone with a hearing loss** may not be able to hear an emergency signal or know that you are speaking to him or her.

◆ Be sure to face the person when you are speaking so that he or she may read your lips.

◆ Explain the emergency system, and tell guests what to *look for*, if they cannot hear signals.

◆ Simple, repetitive phrases will be most easily understood.

Remember, disabled persons **don't** want pity, and they don't want special treatment: they simply wish to be treated like everybody else. If you communicate in an open and friendly manner and without "talking down" to them, you will help them enjoy your facility in a safe manner.

Medic Alert Tags

Some disabled persons will wear Medic Alert tags, which can help you determine needs. Most individuals who wear such tags will (of their own accord) discuss their condition and necessary precautions with you. If an individual who wears such a tag has not discussed it with you, it is perfectly acceptable for you to ask for such information.

When and How to Rescue

Knowing when to rescue a disabled person is essential. No lifeguard likes to do a "bogus" rescue, but it is worse to fail to recognize a real need for help. Most disabled persons will know and use the same distress signals other people use: those distress signs you have already learned. These signs include:

- Thrashing arms and inability to raise head for air.
- Facial expression indicating fear or distress.
- Drastic change in movement patterns.
- Lack of movement.
- Obvious inability to regain footing after losing balance.

The rescue techniques taught in this course can all be effectively used to assist most disabled persons. The obvious exceptions are situations in which:

- The disabled person cannot **see** the equipment.
- The disabled person cannot **hear** your instructions or encouragements.
- The disabled person cannot **grasp** or **hold** the equipment.

In such instances, you **use what works**: use a technique that will give you control of the disabled guest and the situation. You can explain your actions after the rescue.

Learning about disabilities and how they affect a person in the water will help you recognize problems and deal more effectively with safety issues. If possible, learn first hand about the disability by asking disabled guests to tell you what their limitations are. Open, friendly communication will allow you to learn, and let disabled guests know that you are concerned about their safety and enjoyment of your facility.

LIFEGUARDING WATERPARKS AND SPECIAL FACILITIES

Moving water, waves, slides, and other aquatic attractions present special lifeguarding and safety needs. Every skill and technique you have learned in this course has been designed around meeting these special needs. However, there are additional considerations you need to be aware of before lifeguarding a special facility.

Each facility is different, with its own special safety needs. This is why you will spend in-service time becoming familiar with the attractions where you will be lifeguarding. As you train at your special facility, you will learn how to further adapt some of your skills to meet the needs of the attraction. For example:

- Time your compact jump into a wave pool so that you hit the wave at its peak, not the trough. The trough is the low point between waves where the water is shallow.
- When making an assist or rescue, attempt to face the distressed guest away from the direction of currents, flumes, or waves. This will allow you to use the moving water for support.

◆ Know how to activate your E-stop and/or your stop dispatch signals.

◆ Be aware of the unique characteristics of special facilities and how they may affect the way you lifeguard.

Waterparks and special facilities usually:

◆ Attract new guests daily.

◆ Attract great numbers of guests.

◆ Have a large lifeguard staff.

◆ Have multi-attraction facilities.

◆ Have frequent rescues on a daily basis.

◆ Attract greater media exposure.

◆ Attract recreational swimmers.

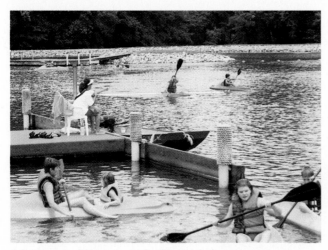

Adapt your skills to your facility and guests: protected lakefront.

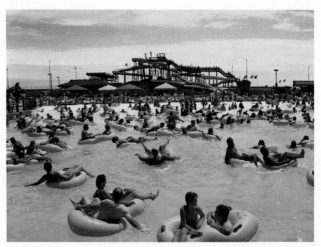

Adapt your skills to your facility and guests: waterpark.

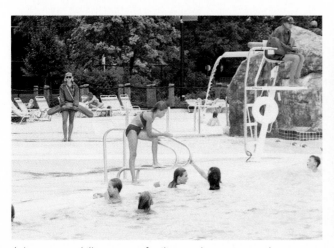

Adapt your skills to your facility and guests: pool.

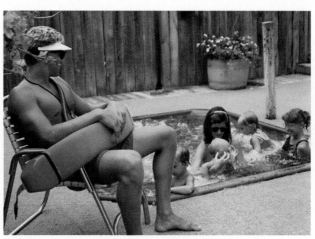

Adapt your skills to your facility and guests: spa.

LIFEGUARDING POOLS

Pool lifeguarding presents its own unique challenges because of the nature of the guests and the facility. Pool facilities usually:

◆ Attract returning local guests.

◆ Have few or no rescues per season.

◆ Offer diversified aquatic programs for guests with a wide range of ages and abilities.

◆ Attract all types of swimmers for various reasons.

A major challenge of lifeguarding at a pool facility is maintaining professionalism and diligence. The familiar guests whom you see each day, the relaxed environment, and the lack of frequent rescues can all lead to a feeling of security and a sense that "nothing will ever happen here." Remember that many drownings occur each year in guarded flatwater pools. Many times this can be attributed to the boredom or lack of attentiveness of the lifeguard. A swimming pool is generally not as exciting or active as a waterpark, and it is easy to let your concentration wander. Allowing yourself to have a laid-back attitude, even for a few minutes, can be the biggest mistake you will ever make.

LIFEGUARDING SPECIAL EVENTS

Ellis & Associates client facilities must maintain the 10/20 Protection Rule and have a lifeguard on duty anytime the pool is in use, regardless of the activity. The only exception is if an outside organization is renting the facility and providing for their own safety. (A written agreement to that effect must be on file.)

As a result, you may find yourself lifeguarding a wide range of special events or activities. Some of these events may include: swim meets, swim shows, triathlons, swim practices, waterpolo games, surfing competitions, lifeguard competitions, swim lessons, or water fitness classes.

Each of these events will require special scanning techniques to maintain the 10/20 Protection Rule. It is very important that you understand the nature of the activity you will be lifeguarding before it begins so you can be prepared. Before the event, find out:

◆ The number of swimmers who are expected.

◆ If the event is continuous or will have staggered participation.

◆ If your usual lifeguard position will be changed or relocated.

◆ Who the person in charge of the event will be.

◆ If there are any special considerations you need to be aware of.

LIFEGUARDING PROTECTED LAKEFRONTS

The design of the lakefront will determine if it is necessary for you to guard from a boat, rescue board, or the shore. You will spend in-service time practicing the use of different skills and equipment that may be unique to your facility.

In a lake you have no visibility beneath the water, so your attention must be entirely focused on guests on the surface. If guests slip quietly beneath the surface, you will not be able to see them and their disappearance may not be known until someone reports them missing.

If you are guarding at a lakefront, you will need to be trained in the use of masks, fins, and snorkles. You and your backup lifeguards must be able to conduct a bottom search of the entire area and recover a guest on the bottom within 3 minutes. Lifeguarding a protected lakefront can be a very difficult and demanding task.

Lakefronts usually:

◆ Attract returning local guests and new guests.

◆ Have changing features that cannot be controlled.

◆ Attract all ages and types of guests.

◆ Have frequent rescues.

◆ Have poor water clarity, which reduces visibility.

◆ Have a higher incidence of intoxicated guests.

◆ Frequently have no fee to enter, which limits control of users.

◆ Require that lifeguards use special equipment.

Lakefronts will be of a variety of designs. The more enclosed the area, the easier it is to guard. The more open the area, the more difficult it is to guard. The bottom contours, debris, and subsurface grass create changing and dangerous conditions. It will be important that you inspect the lakefront swimming area on a daily basis and make adjustments as needed. As the season progresses, and the water level of the lake drops, guard chairs may need to be relocated closer to the new water line.

REVIEW QUESTIONS

1. List three types of disabilities and how they may affect that person at your facility.

   a.

   b.

   c.

2. List two strategies for dealing with a person with a mental impairment.

   a.

   b.

3. List two strategies for dealing with a person who is blind.

   a.

   b.

4. List two strategies for dealing with a person who is deaf.

   a.

   b.

5. List two strategies for dealing with a person who is physically disabled.

   a.

   b.

6. List two strategies for dealing with a person who has a speech impairment.

   a.

   b.

7. T   F   When rescuing a disabled person, "use what works" if he or she cannot see your equipment, hear your instructions, or grasp or hold the equipment.

8. List three differences between waterparks and public swimming facilities:

Waterparks	Public Swimming Facilities
a.	a.
b.	b.
c.	c.

9. A major challenge of lifeguarding at a pool facility is maintaining

   a.

   b.

10. In making a rescue or assist in currents or flumes, face the distressed guest _____ from the direction of the currents to use the moving water for support.

11. T   F   Time your jump into a wave pool so you hit the wave at its trough.

12. T   F   The 10/20 Protection Rule does not need to be maintained at special events such as swim meets, swim lessons, lifeguard competitions, water shows, etc.

13. T   F   Lifeguards at a protected lakefront must be able to do a complete bottom search in 3 minutes.

SKILL SHEET 22

Adapting Lifeguarding Skills

1
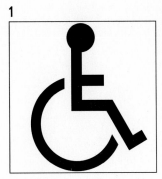
Disabled.

2
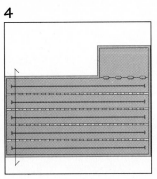
Protected lakefront.

3
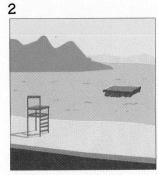
Waterpark.

4
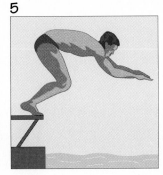
Pools.

5
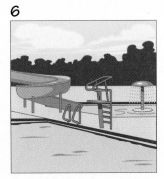
Special events.

6
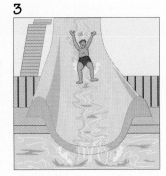
Special features.

KEY POINTS:	CRITICAL THINKING:
◆ Be flexible. ◆ Make it work. ◆ Remember the 10/20 Protection Rule.	1. For each situation above, think of how you would have to adapt your lifeguarding skills. 2. How do you determine if a situation is being managed for the best possible safety?

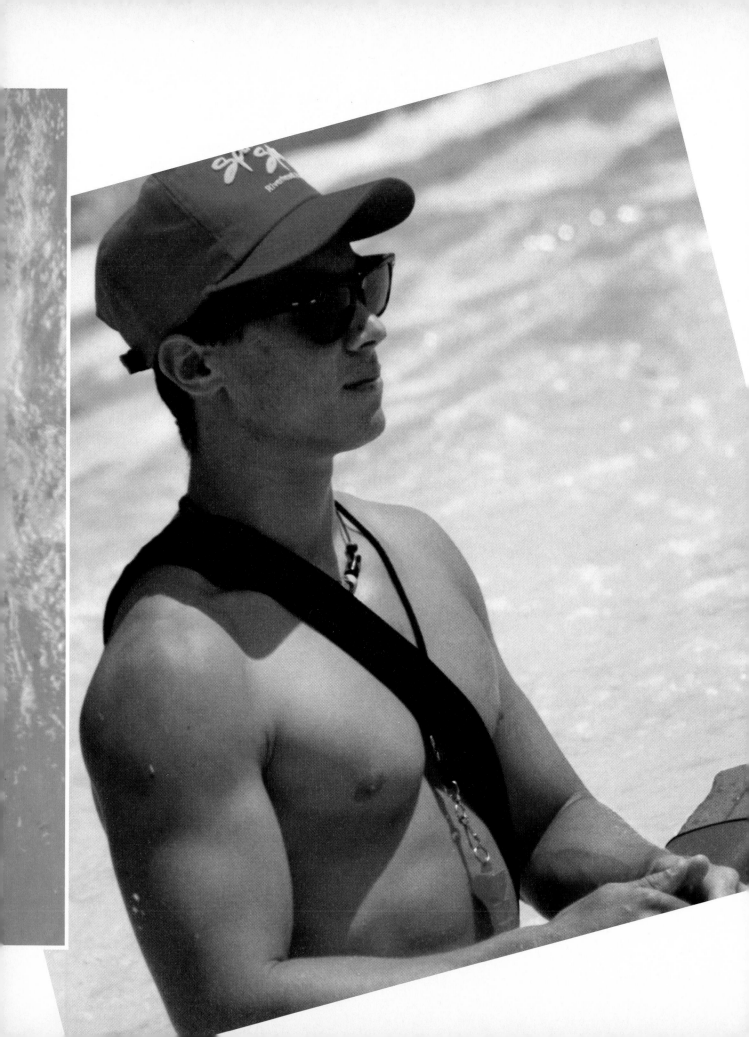

CHAPTER

13

How Will I Be Held Accountable for My Skill Level and Professionalism?

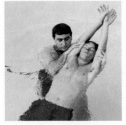

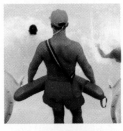

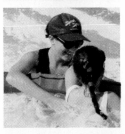

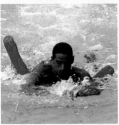

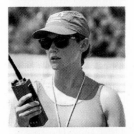

CHAPTER OBJECTIVES

After completing the chapter and related water work, the lifeguard candidate should be able to:

1. Understand the concept of and reasons for the auditing process.
2. Describe how an audit is conducted.
3. Identify ways to guarantee a successful audit performance.

The National Pool and Waterpark Lifeguard (NPWLTP) Training Program equips you to perform professional lifeguarding by anticipating, recognizing, and managing aquatic emergencies. You provide the most critical, frontline component in a comprehensive, professional water safety and risk management system coordinated by Ellis & Associates.

Safety records and statistics document the fact that facilities implementing the complete Ellis & Associates system provide the highest standard of aquatic care. As a result, the NPWL license has become the "standard of care" in the aquatic industry.

Ellis & Associates, your facility management, and your facilities insurance company are all interested in preventing losses and in providing a safe environment for guests. They will work together in the total risk management program.

A major component of the Ellis & Associates risk management program is the independent audits. This means that an Ellis & Associates staff person will come, unannounced, into your facility to observe how well you and other lifeguards are functioning in normal day-to-day as well as emergency situations.

An auditor does not come into your facility to find out everything you are doing wrong. Instead, an auditor will randomly choose (ahead of arrival) a specific location to observe. What the auditor will determine is: if during that particular time of observation, an aquatic emergency had occurred, would the lifeguard have been able to anticipate, recognize, and manage the incident?

This means that your scanning skills and ability to maintain the 10/20 Protection Rule will be observed and documented. Your professionalism and diligence will be evaluated, along with your personal safety responsibilities. You may also be asked to manage a simulated aquatic emergency to document your rescue and technical skills.

You need to maintain all of your skills at "test ready" levels at all times. Your performance will become a part of your facilities risk management documents in both written report and video report form. Your audit score will also determine the safety award category for your facility. Professional lifeguards perform well during audits, because they perform well every minute they are on the job.

REVIEW QUESTIONS

1. T F   The National Pool and Waterpark Lifeguard License has become the standard of care in the aquatic industry.

2. T F   As a lifeguard, you are one component in a total risk management program at your facility.

3. When an auditor visits your facility, he or she will document if you could:

   a. _____ , b. _____ , and c. _____ an aquatic emergency during that specific time of observation.

4. Part of an audit will also include documenting your level of

a.

b.

5. T   F   Professional lifeguards perform well during audits, because they perform well every minute they are on the job.

SKILL SHEET 23

Audit Performance
Do You Meet, Exceed, or Fail Standards?

1

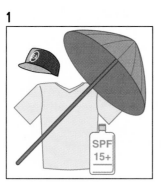

Sun Protection
Two or more barriers
Sunscreen SPF 15+

2

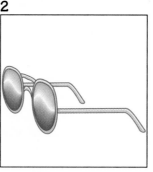

Sunglasses
100% UV

3

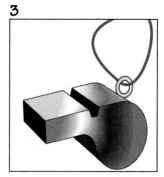

Whistle
Blow firmly
No twirling

4

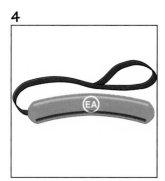

Rescue Tube
Hold professionally
Gather strap

5

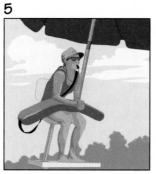

Posture
Feet flat
Shoulders forward
Sit straight

6

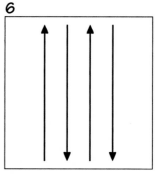

Scanning
10/20 Protection Rule
Have pattern
Know zone

7

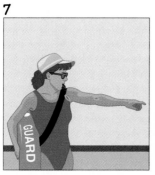

Communication
Golden Rule

8

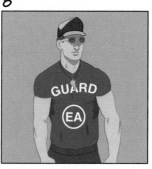

Professionalism and Uniform
Stand out

9

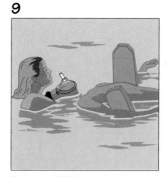

Rescue Skills
In-service often
Always "rescue ready"

KEY POINTS:

- Practice skills.
- Be responsible.
- Be mature.
- Do your job well.
- Be a professional lifeguard.

CRITICAL THINKING:

For each of the categories above, what would you consider:

- Exceeding standard?
- Meeting standard?
- Failing standard?

Appendices

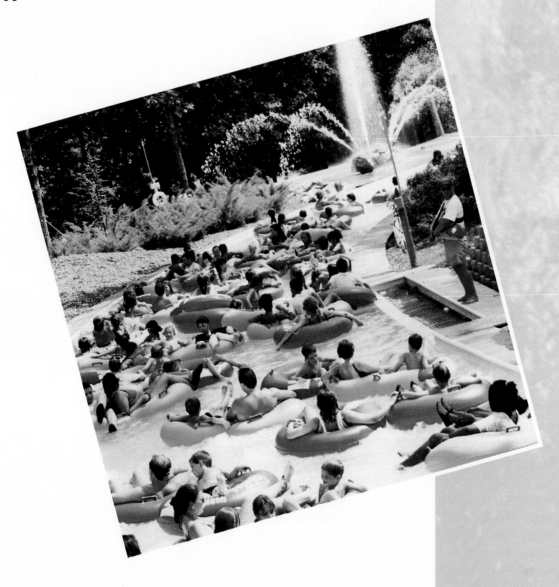

SAMPLE
■ RESCUE FLOW (ACTIVE) ■

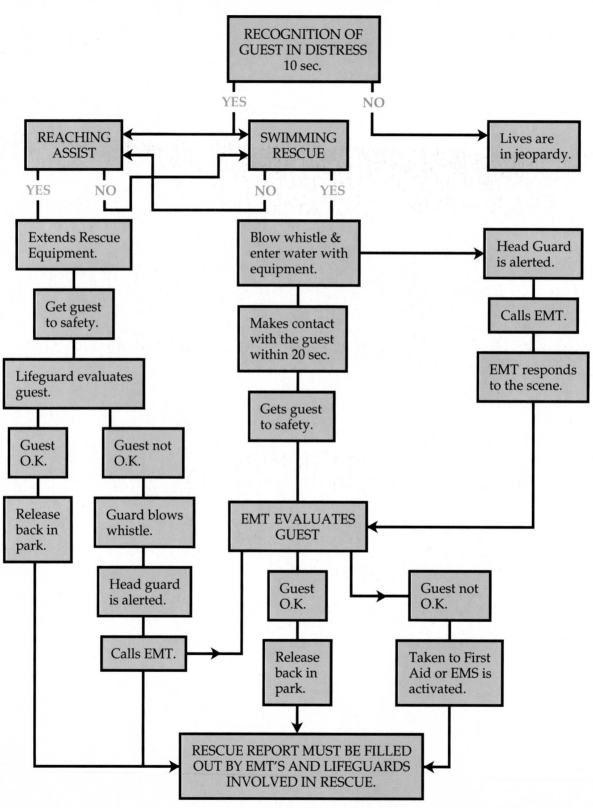

SAMPLE
■ RESCUE FLOW (PASSIVE) ■

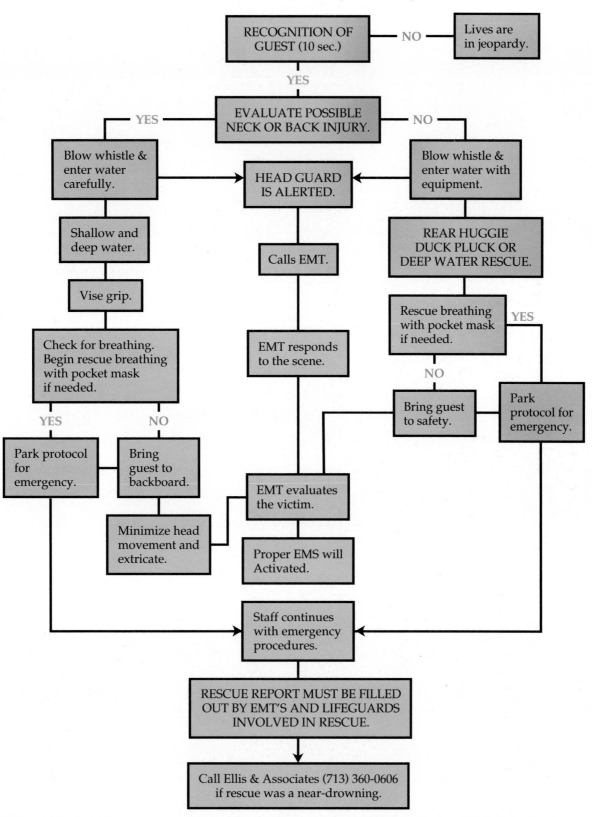

National Pool and Waterpark Lifeguard Training Program
Lifeguard License Transfer Application

Last Name			First Name			Middle Name

Address			City		State	Zip Code

Date of Birth		Age	Home Telephone Number

Social Security Number		Sex	Work Telephone Number

INSTRUCTIONS:

This form is to be utilized by licensed NPWLTP lifeguards who desire to work for a nonclient aquatic facility. In order to receive NPWLTP authorization to work for a nonclient aquatic facility, the lifeguard must submit this transfer request to ELLIS & ASSOCIATES after complying with the NPWLTP requirements set forth below.

1. Type or print all requested information in the shaded areas of this form.

2. Submit the completed form along with a $25 transfer processing fee to ELLIS & ASSOCIATES.

3. Read, sign, and submit the nonclient lifeguarding agreement in the NPWLTP textbook.

4. Have the nonclient facility operator (employer) read, sign, and submit the "Nonclient Facility Agreement" in the NPWLTP textbook supplement to ELLIS & ASSOCIATES.

NOTE: NPWLTP lifeguard licenses are only valid when you are working for a client aquatic facility of ELLIS & ASSOCIATES. Nonclient aquatic facilities must meet all criteria as set forth in the "Nonclient Facility Agreement" before you will receive NPWLTP approval to work at a nonclient aquatic facility. Failure to receive NPWLTP authorization prior to working at a nonclient aquatic facility violates the terms and conditions of your NPWLTP license and terminates the licensing agreement.

When was your most recent NPWLTP license issued?

Where was your NPWLTP course conducted?

Who was your NPWLTP course instructor?

What is your NPWLTP license number?

What is the name, address, telephone number, and operator manager of the nonclient facility?

Return to: Ellis & Associates, 3506 Spruce Park Circle, Kingwood, Texas 77345
Telephone: (713) 360-0606 FAX Number: (713) 360-0869

Review Question Answers

INTRODUCTION AND CHAPTER 1 REVIEW ANSWERS

1. A shallow water lifeguard operates and protects guests in water that is 4 feet or less in depth.
2. The license is valid for 1 year.
3. There are several areas of emphasis of the NPWLTP that include:

   a. Professional lifeguarding.
   b. Frequency of rescues.
   c. Rescue tube rescues.
   d. Total risk management, including audits.
   e. Techniques and training based on actual data.
   f. Integrating CPR and lifeguard first responder skills.

4. False. Dry drowning only occurs about 20 percent of the time.
5. False. To aspirate water means to "draw by suction" water into the lungs. To asphyxiate means to suffocate.
6. True. Rescue the guest if necessary, then assess ABC's as taught in CPR.
7. True. Guests may experience a dry drowning either in or out of the water.
8. True. Individuals, especially children, may not always follow the "stages" of wet drowning.
9. Guests who would be considered high risk might include:

   a. Children between the ages of 7 and 12.
   b. Non swimmers or poor swimmers.
   c. Parents in the water with their small children.
   d. An intoxicated individual.
   e. People with unusual or extreme body proportions.
   f. The elderly.
   g. Someone wearing a lifejacket.
   h. Guests wearing clothes.

10. Running is the leading cause of guest injury.
11. Most rescues occur midday.
12. True. All swimmers are at risk at your facility. An accident can happen to anyone.
13. False. A guest on the bottom may be very difficult to see, not easy.
14. True. Guests can be conscious on the bottom and still need rescuing.
15. False. Scanning patterns *should* be changed to prevent boredom.
16. True. It is important to look professional and maintain the 10/20 Protection Rule when rotating.
17. The 10/20 Protection Rule allows you 10 seconds to see and recognize an aquatic emergency, and 20 seconds to perform a rescue and begin management of the situation.
18. False. You *should scan the entire* **physical area** of the zone you are responsible for, *even if there are no swimmers* in that part of the facility.

CHAPTER 2 REVIEW ANSWERS

1. The emergency action system is activated by one long whistle blast.
2. The lifeguard to the rescuer's **left** covers the zone when a lifeguard is making a rescue.
3. Matching:

__(C)__ one short whistle	gain swimmer attention
__(G)__ raised fist	lifeguard needs help
__(A)__ two long whistles	major emergency
__(H)__ crossed arms	stop dispatch
__(D)__ tapping head	watch my area
__(F)__ one long whistle	rescue in progress
__(B)__ pointing	give direction
__(E)__ thumbs up	resume activity

4. What should be posted next to the telephone?

    a. Telephone numbers of emergency services.
    b. Clear directions to your facility.
    c. Number of Poison Control Center.

5. The difference between an assist and a rescue is that an assist can be done while still maintaining the 10/20 Protection Rule.

6. Name three things you could use to make an extension assist.

    a. Reaching pole.
    b. Body part (arm, leg, etc.).
    c. Rescue equipment (rescue tube, ring buoy, etc.).

7. When making an assist or a rescue, it is important to reassure the guest by talking to them.

8. False. The rescue tube is a **mandatory** piece of equipment, not optional.

CHAPTER 3 REVIEW ANSWERS

1. True. The difference between a **distressed swimmer rescue** and a **near drowning rescue** is that in a near drowning the guest is unconscious and successfully revived by the lifeguard, and a distressed swimmer is rescued before the situation becomes life-threatening.

2. False. The compact jump entry is performed with the legs together, not apart.

3. True. In order for a front drive to be successful, you must keep your arms straight and keep driving by kicking as hard as you can.

4. True. Active guests in distress can be approached from the front or the rear.

5. False. Communication between lifeguards in a two-guard rescue **is** important.

6. It is important to always try to grab a guest underneath the armpit, as soon as possible, when assisting a guest to prevent injuring the shoulder.

CHAPTER 4 REVIEW ANSWERS

1. List three things you may have to do to adapt a rear huggie for use with an unconscious guest.

    a. Pull the guest back onto the tube.
    b. Kick, while pulling back.
    c. Make sure the tube is under the guest's upper back.

2. It is important to immediately start rescue breathing in the water because the shorter the amount of time a guest has been without air, the better the chances for survival. The first minute is critical.

3. True. Universal Precautions means to treat **all** body fluids as if they are contaminated and take measures to protect yourself from exposure to them.

4. True. Placing an unconscious guest on the rescue tube, with the tube under the back, is usually an ideal open airway position.

5. Four reasons for using a pocket mask in the water are:

    a. It forms a seal to prevent water from entering the guest's mouth and blocking the airway.
    b. It protects the lifeguard from the guest's body fluids.

    c. It protects the guest from the lifeguard's body fluids.
    d. It allows rescue breathing to be performed during the crucial time when the guest needs air instead of having to wait until the guest is removed from the water.

6. True. When removing an unconscious guest from the water, it is important to do it quickly, with minimal risk of injury to the guest or to you.

7. The rate of rescue breathing in the water for an adult is one breath every 5 seconds.

8. The rate of rescue breathing in the water for a child is one breath every 3 seconds.

9. True. Another word for removal is **extrication.**

10. True. A method of removing an unconscious guest that is both quick and safe is to use a backboard, without the straps or head piece, using the two-guard technique.

CHAPTER 5 REVIEW ANSWERS

1. True. CPR skills are easy to learn, and if practiced often, easy to recall.

2. Put the following steps in the primary survey in order:

    __1__ Shake and shout, "Are you OK?"

    __2__ If the guest does not respond, call for help.

    __3__ Head tilt-chin lift, or jaw thrust.

    __4__ Look, listen, and feel.

    __5__ Give two full breaths.

    __6__ Check for pulse.

3. If a guest has a pulse, but is not breathing, you should begin rescue breathing at the correct rate for an adult, infant or child, and check the pulse again every few minutes.

4. If a guest is breathing on his or her own, you should place the guest in the recovery position and monitor breathing.

5. False. An infant's pulse should **not** be checked at their carotid artery in the neck; it should be checked at the brachial artery in the upper arm, for 5–10 seconds.

6. True. If a breath does not go in, reposition the head and try again.

7. If repositioning the head does not open an obstructed airway in an adult or child, you should then give __5__ abdominal thrusts.

8. Match the rescue breathing rates with the type of guest:

    __C__ Infant   1 breath every 3 seconds

    __B__ Child   1 breath every 3 seconds

    __A__ Adult   1 breath every 5 seconds

9. True. Counting for the rescue breathing rate should be done out loud, and with the count of one one-thousand, two one-thousand, three one-thousand, four one-thousand **breathe** for an adult.

10. True. For a person who has an obstructed airway and is conscious, the Heimlich maneuver of grasping around the guest from behind and performing quick, upward abdominal thrusts until the object is dislodged or they become unconscious is the best method.

CHAPTER 6 REVIEW ANSWERS

1. False. It **is** important to talk to a guest with a spinal injury, because he or she will probably be **conscious,** not unconscious.
2. True. It is your job to prevent further injury to the guest until EMS arrives.
3. True. Guests with head or spinal injuries are likely to suffer hypothermia more quickly than usual because of the trauma to their system and should be removed from the water as quickly as possible and kept warm.
4. True. The vise grip is a rescue technique used for a guest with a suspected spinal injury . . . with the tube on top of the water, without the tube if a guest is on the bottom.
5. False. An **ease-in** entry is used if a spinal injury is suspected, not a compact jump.
6. True. You must evaluate each situation carefully to determine if you should suspect a spinal injury, based on the guest's location, activity, and depth of the water.

CHAPTER 7 REVIEW ANSWERS

1. True. Many times, guests may be submerged just a couple of feet, but they are unable to get to the surface.
2. To help keep you from pulling yourself into the guest or pulling yourself over the top of the rescue tube you can:

   a. Steady yourself on the rescue tube with one hand.
   b. Push the tube underwater as you make your grab.
   c. Push the tube with one hand, while pulling the guest up with the other.

CHAPTER 8 REVIEW ANSWERS (SPECIAL FACILITY AND POOL LIFEGUARD CANDIDATES ONLY)

1. True. In a deep water rescue, your rescue tube will help you bring even a very large guest to the surface.
2. When surface diving to the bottom, you should descend <u>feet</u> first.
3. After feet first surface diving to the bottom, you should position yourself <u>behind</u> the guest.
4. If a guest is submerged in deep water and is **conscious,** you will pull the tube <u>in front</u> of the guest's body when you break the surface of the water. If the guest is **unconscious,** you will pull the tube <u>behind</u> the guest's body to place the head in an open airway position.

CHAPTER 9 REVIEW ANSWERS

1. For each of the physical conditions listed, name one action you can take to minimize the effects.

   a. Dehydration <u>drink plenty of fluids.</u>
   b. Skin cancer <u>use sunscreen plus barriers such as umbrella, clothes, hat.</u>
   c. Cataracts <u>wear sunglasses that screen out 100% UV rays.</u>

2. True. Standard of Care refers to the skills and care that would normally be known and done by others working as professional lifeguards in the same position.
3. True. If you are involved in a lawsuit, it could take many years and be financially draining.
4. False. In-service training should be held 4 hours per month, not 1 hour.
5. True. The best way to protect yourself from legal liability is to be attentive, conscientious, efficient, and skilled.
6. List a minimum of four things you can do to reduce the emotional effects of being involved in a near-drowning rescue.

   a. Get in the water and have a physical workout.
   b. Remember that being questioned is necessary, just relax.
   c. Fill out your report accurately.
   d. Be prepared for possibly misleading media coverage—don't let it bother you.
   e. Put the incident behind you—you will never forget it, but you don't have to keep thinking about it.
   f. Keep up your regular, familiar schedule. Keep up school and job.
   g. Be supportive of other members of your lifeguard team.
   h. Take advantage of trained individuals who can help you deal with the stress.

CHAPTER 10 REVIEW ANSWERS

1. True. Basic first responder skills, if not performed, could lead to additional injury and possible death for the guest.
2. True. Life-threatening emergencies for the lifeguard first responder are those that compromise the guest's airway, breathing, or circulation in any manner, including those situations in which massive bleeding is found.
3. False. As a lifeguard first responder, your safety comes **first,** not second.
4. True. Guests can have a pulse but not be breathing.
5. True. Guests without a pulse will not be breathing.
6. You perform a secondary survey only after the primary survey has been completed, and any problems with airway, breathing, circulation, or hemorrhaging have been controlled.
7. In a secondary survey, you are looking for any additional injuries by feeling head to toe while asking about complaints, history, and other information. You relate all this information to the EAS/EMS team when they arrive.

8. Match the symptoms with the type of burn:

    __C__ First degree   Red skin, slight swelling, pain.

    __A__ Second degree   Blisters, pain.

    __B__ Third degree   Slight pain at burn site, multicolored skin.

9. Match the type of burn with emergency treatment:

    __A__ First degree   Place area in cool water until pain stops.

    __C__ Second degree   Cover area with moist, clean sheets.

    __B__ Third degree   Maintain airway, cover with clean cloth, transport to hospital.

10. In addition to heat or flame, list three other sources of burns and how to treat them:

    a. Chemical. Brush off if dry, flush with water until pain stops.

    b. Electrical. Remove source, check ABC's, treat as heat burns.

    c. Lightning. Check ABC's, treat as heat burns.

11. Match the symptoms with the type of heat emergency:

    __C__ Heat cramps   Leg, abdomen, calf cramps plus dizziness.

    __B__ Heat exhaustion   Cool, sweaty, pale skin; nausea, headache.

    __A__ Heat stroke   Hot skin, rapid pulse, tremors, confusion.

12. True. Heat stroke is a life-threatening condition.
13. True. Sprains, strains, dislocations, and fractures should be cared for only after doing a primary survey and finding everything OK.
14. True. Bleeding that is "squirting" comes from arteries and must be controlled immediately.
15. Matching:

    __(D)__ Direct pressure   First method of controlling bleeding.

    __(F)__ Elevation   Along with direct pressure, the second stage of controlling bleeding.

    __(G)__ Pressure points   Places around the body where an artery can be pressed against a bone to slow the flow of blood.

    __(B)__ Contusion   Bruise.

    __(A)__ Avulsion   Skin flap injury.

    __(E)__ Universal Precautions   Protecting yourself from contact with body fluids.

16. True. To treat for fainting, monitor the guest's ABC's, look for any active bleeding, elevate legs, loosen restrictive clothing, and place in recovery position until the guest feels better.
17. False. There are many different causes of seizures, **but each is treated the same, regardless of the cause.**
18. True. Never force anything into the mouth of a seizuring guest, attempt to restrain him or her, or give food or drink.
19. The type of shock that occurs when the body has a severe allergic reaction is called anaphylactic shock.
20. If a guest has been stung or bitten by an insect and is exhibiting signs of a reaction, you should activate EAS/EMS and find out if the guest has any medication to control the reaction.
21. When treating a soft tissue wound, your role as a lifeguard first responder is to:

    a. Control bleeding.
    b. Reduce the chance for infection.

22. True. When treating for hypovolemic shock, keep the guest warm, with elevated legs, but do not overheat.
23. True. Lifeguard first responders are not a replacement for the EAS/EMS professionals—activate the EAS/EMS early.

CHAPTER 11 REVIEW ANSWERS

1. Being professional means: (e)

    a. Being in full uniform, easily identified and neat and clean.
    b. Being pleasant to guests and staff at all times.
    c. Paying attention to placement and condition of your rescue equipment.

2. List three things that might lessen the number of times you have to enforce a rule.

    a. Understand and explain the rules.
    b. Enforce rules uniformly.
    c. Use a positive approach.
    d. Know where rules are posted.
    e. Refer problems to your superior.
    f. Remember the Golden Rule.

3. What is the Golden Rule?

    Treat people like you would like to be treated.

4. List three things that will help you control a crowd.

    a. Keep yourself calm.
    b. Speak loudly and clearly.
    c. Give precise, simple directions.
    d. Speak with authority.

5. False. **All** rescues need documentation, not just near drownings.
6. Working as a lifeguard means that you (f. All of the above):

    a. Should expect to have regular in-service training.
    b. Could be physically injured.
    c. Might have to work in bad weather conditions.

d. Might have to perform unrelated duties at your facility.

e. Will be expected to maintain professional standards.

CHAPTER 12 REVIEW ANSWERS

1. List three types of disabilities and how they may affect that person at your facility:

   a. Physically disabled—movement or balance problems.

   b. Mentally disabled—may not understand.

   c. Sensory impairments—may communicate differently.

2. List two strategies for dealing with a person with a mental impairment.

   a. Repeat rules, or remind them.

   b. Keep explanations short and simple.

3. List two strategies for dealing with a person who is blind.

   a. Mention landmarks and "sound" marks.

   b. Give verbal warning before you touch the person.

4. List two strategies for dealing with a person who is deaf.

   a. Face the person so they may read your lips.

   b. Explain what to **look for** if the emergency system is activated.

5. List two strategies for dealing with a person who is physically disabled.

   a. Know that they may have difficulties in the wave pool because of less effective movement.

   b. Offer them a lifejacket to aid with buoyancy.

6. List two strategies for dealing with a person who has a speech impairment.

   a. Be sure to find a way to understand them if they are trying to ask a qustion; try writing, a symbol board, or an interpreter.

   b. Be an assertive listener.

7. True. When rescuing a disabled person, "use what works" if they cannot see your equipment, hear your instructions, or grasp or hold the equipment.

8. List three differences between waterparks and public swimming facilities:

   Waterparks
   a. Attract new guests daily.
   b. Attract great numbers of guests.
   c. Have a large lifeguard staff.
   d. Have multiattraction facilities.
   e. Have frequent rescues on daily basis.
   f. Attract great media exposure.
   g. Attract recreational swimmers.

Public Swimming Facilities:
   a. Attract returning local guests.
   b. Have few rescues.
   c. Have a small lifeguard staff.
   d. Offer diversified programs.
   e. Attract all types of swimmers.

9. A major challenge of lifeguarding at a pool facility is maintaining:

   a. Professionalism.

   b. Diligence.

10. In making a rescue or assist in currents or flumes, face the distressed guest away from the direction of the currents to use the moving water for support.

11. False. Time your jump into a wave pool so you hit the wave **peak**, not at its trough.

12. False. The 10/20 Protection Rule **does** need to be maintained at special events such as swim meets, swim lessons, lifeguard competitions, water shows, etc. There are no exceptions to the 10/20 Protection Rule.

13. True. Lifeguards at a protected lakefront must be able to do a complete bottom search in 3 minutes.

CHAPTER 13 REVIEW ANSWERS

1. True. The National Pool & Waterpark Lifeguard License has become the standard of care in the aquatic industry.

2. True. As a lifeguard, you are one component in a total risk management program at your facility.

3. When an auditor visits your facility, he or she will document if you could:

   a. Anticipate.

   b. Recognize.

   c. Manage.

   an aquatic emergency during that specific time of observation.

4. Part of an audit will also include documenting your level of:

   a. Professionalism.

   b. Diligence.

5. True. Professional lifeguards perform well during audits, because they perform well every minute they are on the job.

Glossary of Key Terms

10/20 Protection Rule   Allowing a lifeguard 10 seconds to recognize an aquatic emergency and another 20 seconds to perform a rescue and begin care. (Chapter 1)

Abdominal Thrust   Pushing upward on the abdomen to remove a foreign body obstruction and open the airway. (Chapter 5)

Abrasion   An open wound from a scrape that damages the surface of the skin. (Chapter 10)

Airway Management   Keeping open the passage through which air goes into the lungs. (Chapters 4, 5, 10)

Anaphylactic Shock   A type of shock that occurs when the body has a severe allergic reaction. (Chapter 10)

Assist   To help a distressed swimmer while still being able to maintain the 10/20 Protection Rule in the zone. (Chapter 2)

Audit   The process through which lifeguards are held accountable for maintaining their skills and professionalism at "test-ready" levels at all times. (Chapter 13)

Avulsion   An open wound with a portion of the skin or tissue torn away from the body. (Chapter 10)

Backboard   A rigid board with straps to secure the body and a device to secure the head. It is used to remove a guest with a suspected spinal injury from the water while minimizing the movement of the body and the head. It is also used without straps to quickly and safely remove an unconscious guest from the water. (Chapter 6)

Blood-borne Pathogen   Viruses or other disease organisms that are carried by the blood. (Chapters 4, 10)

Cardiopulmonary   Referring to the heart (cardio) and lungs (pulmonary). (Chapter 5)

Compact Jump   An entry into the water from a height keeping the rescue tube up under the armpits, feet flat, knees slightly bent. It is designed to minimize the risk of injury to the lifeguard while allowing for speed in initiating a rescue. (Chapter 3)

CPR   A combination of chest compressions and rescue breathing used to help sustain oxygen to the brain via the lungs until EMS arrives. It is used for someone who is not breathing and does not have a pulse. (Chapter 5)

Crowd Control   Giving directions or controlling the behavior of a large group of people at one time. (Chapter 11)

Deep Water Rescue   A rescue in which the guest in distress is below arm's reach. (Chapter 8)

Dehydration   Loss of water in the body. (Chapter 10)

Disability   A condition that takes away the normal ability to do something. (Chapter 12)

Distress   Being unable to maintain a position on top of the water, or being unable to make progress to safety without assistance. (Chapters 1, 2, 3)

Drowning   Death caused by A) a fluid in the lungs or B) a laryngospasm. (Chapter 1)

Duck Pluck   A rescue technique used to bring a person who is just under the surface of the water to the top, using a rescue tube. (Chapter 7)

Emergency Action System   The integration of all the people, equipment, and plans involved in dealing with an emergency, such as the aquatic staff, EMS response team, bystanders, facility administrators, and so on. (Chapter 2)

Emergency Action Plan   A plan written for a specific facility and type of emergency that outlines step-by-step emergency procedures and responsibilities. (Chapter 2)

EMS   The Emergency Medical System that will dispatch trained personnel to an emergency when you call 911 or your local emergency number. (Chapter 2)

Epiglottis   A cartilage behind the tongue which works like a valve over the windpipe. (Chapter 1)

Extrication   Removal. (Chapters 4, 6)

Feet First Surface Dive   A method of propelling the body toward the bottom, feet first, by pushing the water upward with the arms. (Chapter 8)

Foreign Body   An object that causes an obstruction or blockage of a person's airway. (Chapter 5)

Front Drive   A rescue technique used when a guest is actively in distress on top of the water, performed with a rescue tube. (Chapter 3)

Guest Relations   The way in which you treat and respond to guests at your facility. (Chapter 11)

HBV   A virus carried in the blood (blood-borne) that causes Hepatitis B, an incurable disease that affects the liver and is potentially life-threatening. (Chapters 4, 10)

Head Tilt/Chin Lift   Tilting the head back while lifting the chin to open the airway of an unconscious person. (Chapters 5, 10)

Heat Cramps   Cramps in the muscles caused by loss of water and salt from the body due to overexposure to heat. (Chapter 10)

Heat Exhaustion   A heat-related illness that is caused by loss of significant amounts of fluid from perspiration. The symptoms include profuse sweating; fatigue; cool, pale, sweaty skin; nausea/vomiting. (Chapter 10)

Heat Stroke   A life-threatening rise in body temperature due to overexposure to heat and breakdown of the body's temperature control system. It is a life-threatening condition. (Chapter 10)

Hemorrhaging   Massive bleeding. (Chapter 10)

High Risk   Conditions or characteristics that make it more likely for an accident or incident to happen. (Chapter 1)

HIV   A virus carried in the blood (blood-borne) that causes AIDS (Acquired Immune Deficiency Syndrome). (Chapters 4, 10)

Hypothermia   A loss of body heat. (Chapter 10)

Hypovolemic Shock   Inadequate circulation of oxygenated blood to the vital organs, as a result of the body's attempts to recover from severe injury or trauma. (Chapter 10)

Impairment   A condition that takes away from the strength or quality of being able to do something. (Chapter 12)

In-service   Training received after obtaining a lifeguard license and becoming employed at an aquatic facility. (Chapter 11)

Insulin Shock   A condition when a diabetic has too much insulin and/or too little sugar. (Chapter 10)

Jaw Thrust   A method of opening the airway in patients with suspected neck injuries. (Chapters 5, 10)

Laceration   A soft tissue open wound that has ragged or torn edges. (Chapter 10)

Larynx   The upper part of the trachea (windpipe) where the vocal cords are located. (Chapter 1)

Liability   Being legally responsible. (Chapter 9)

Lifeguard First Responder   A lifeguard or aquatic professional who is responsible for activating the EMS when a life-threatening emergency occurs, and managing the emergency with appropriate care until help arrives. (Chapters 4, 5, 10)

Life-threatening   An injury or condition that could cause loss of life if specific care is not given. (Chapter 10)

Musculoskeletal   The muscle and bone systems of the body. (Chapter 10)

Primary Survey   Examining or checking a person to see if they have any life-threatening conditions. (Chapter 10)

Post Incident Stress   The emotional, psychological, and physical stress that can occur after an individual has been involved in a traumatic experience. (Chapter 8)

Professional Image   Giving the impression of responsibility, authority, friendliness, and competency to guests at your facility by the way you look and act. (Chapter 11)

Protected Lakefront   An area of open water that has been sectioned off by buoys, ropes, docks, or boats to control access by guests. (Chapter 12)

Pulse   The verification of a beating heart, achieved by feeling the blood expand and contract in the arteries. (Chapters 5, 10)

Puncture Wound   A wound with little bleeding, caused by a sharp pointed object piercing and entering the skin. (Chapter 10)

Qualifying Questions   Questions asked of an injured guest to determine the possible cause, symptoms, and severity of their injury. (Chapter 6)

Rear Huggie   A rescue technique used for a guest who is on the surface of the water facing away from a rescuer. The technique can be used on an unconscious or conscious guest, and is always performed with a rescue tube. (Chapter 3)

Rescue Tube   A piece of rescue equipment that is always kept between the guest and a rescuer. It is usually made of vinyl-dipped foam for buoyancy, and has a body strap and line. (Chapter 5)

Risk Management   Reducing the likelihood of an accident by controlling the factors that make the situation high risk. (Chapter 1)

Scanning   Moving the eyes across the surface and along the bottom of the zone, within the 10/20 Protection Rule. (Chapter 1)

Seizure   Sudden involuntary changes in the activity level of brain cells usually due to disease, trauma, or overdose/chemical reactions. (Chapter 10)

Shock   A collapse of circulatory function caused by severe injury, blood loss, or disease. (Chapter 10)

Skin Cancer   A cancer caused by sun exposure. (Chapter 9)

Special Event   Any activity that is different from the normal daily routine at a facility. (Chapter 12)

Special Facility   Any facility determined by Ellis & Associates, Inc. to have features that require lifeguards to have specialized training. Examples may include facilities with wave pools, multiple slides, etc. (Chapter 12)

SPF   Sun Protection Factor that indicates the level of protection a sunscreen product gives from ultraviolet rays. (Chapter 8)

Spinal Column   The series of vertebrae forming the backbone of the skeleton. (Chapter 6)

Spinal Cord   The cord of nerve tissue extending through the center of the spinal column. (Chapter 6)

Spinal Injury   Injury to the spinal cord usually caused by a blow to the head, neck, or spine. The compression or severing of the cord can cause paralysis and death. (Chapter 6)

Sprain   Tearing of ligaments from muscles. (Chapter 10)

Standard of Care   The skills and care which would normally be known and done by others working as lifeguards. (Chapter 9)

Strain   Tearing of tendons or muscle. (Chapter 10)

Trough   The low part between two waves. (Chapter 12)

UV Rays   A type of radiation from the sun that produces harmful effects on the body, such as skin cancer.

Variance   Written approval to modify any National Pool and Waterpark Lifeguard Training Program or Ellis & Associates, Inc. policy or procedure. (Chapter 12)

Vertebrae   The bones or segments composing the spinal column. (Chapter 6)

Vise Grip   A rescue technique used to prevent further injury to a guest who is suspected of having suffered a spinal injury. (Chapter 6)

Zone   The area a lifeguard is responsible for scanning and maintaining the 10/20 Protection Rule. (Chapter 1)

Index

Note: Page numbers in *italics* indicate illustrations.